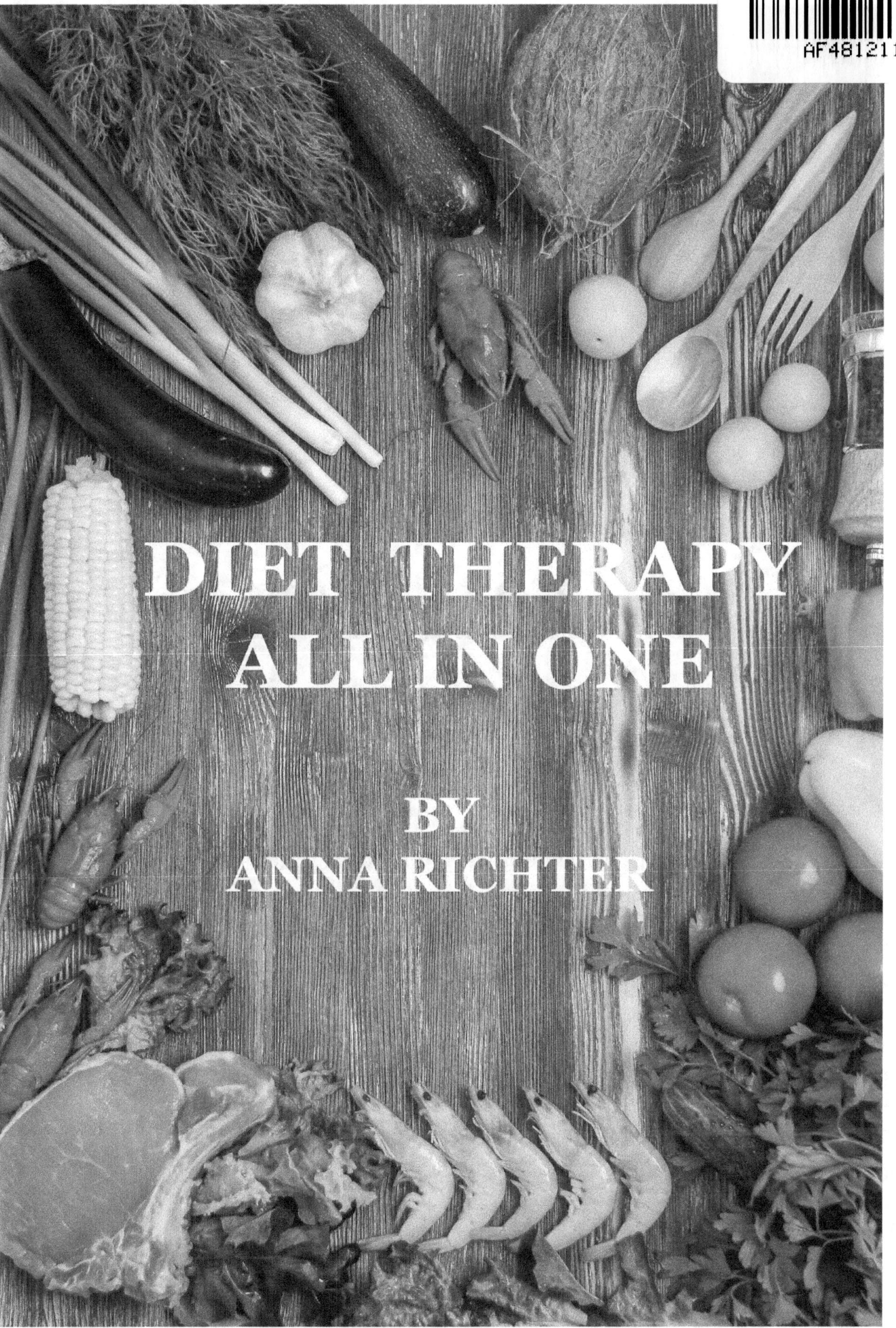

DIET THERAPY
ALL IN ONE
BY
ANNA RICHTER

DIET DESCRIPTIONS,  DIET PLANS, COOKING RECIPES,
MENU RECOMMENDATIONS

# Diet Therapy.
# All in One

FAST DIETS, LOW-CARB DIETS,CLEANSING DIETS,MONO-
DIETS,PROTEIN DIETS

## Anna Richter

ISBN: 9798678635617

# Anna Richter

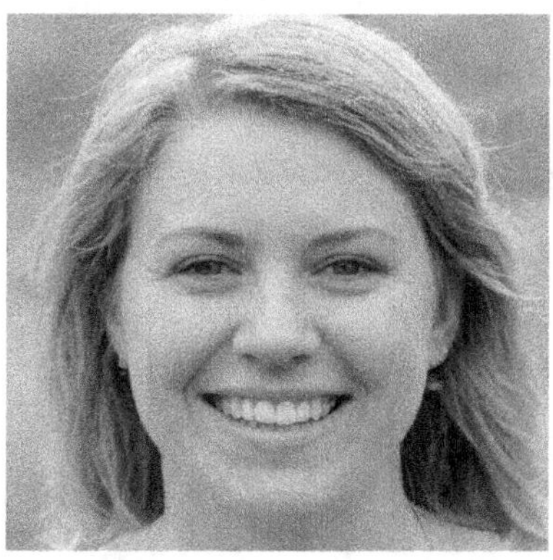

Anna Richter - dietitian, nutritionist, and exercise physiologist with a private nutrition counseling and consulting practice in Berlin, Germany for adolescents, adults, sports teams.

Anna has helped clients with a wide range of nutritional needs enhance their results, improve their life, and make positive lifelong eating and exercise behavior changes. Also she has helped a wide range of clients reach their short and long term nutrition goals to professional athletes, students, and actors, singers , teens, fashion models, and pregnant moms

Anna provides counseling to people with different types of Gestational Diabetes, as well as developing diabetes prevention plans. She works with both pediatrics and adults in the control of their diabetes, using advanced technology to help them achieve optimal blood glucose control.

Anna is a registered wellness consultant and holistic counselor.

# Introduction

This book contains the most popular and effective dietary programs. All diets contain detailed information, the degree of effectiveness, the course of nutrition, divided into different time programs, menus and recipes, as well as recommendations and contraindications.

I divided the diets collected here into several types: fast diets, low-carb diets, detox diets, mono diets, protein diets.

Fast diets, when you need to get back to normal quickly, but you need to understand that in order to achieve quick results, a quick rollback is possible if the exit from the diet was incorrect. On a fast diet in two weeks, you can lose about 7-12 kilograms. The weight loss system is based on controlling the amount of sugar, fat and salt in the diet.

Low-carb diets - allows you to reduce the percentage of body fat, which leads to weight loss and better shape.

Low-carb diets reduce blood glucose levels (if blood sugar is elevated, then it is elevated in the brain, which is extremely dangerous for brain cells, because it contributes to the formation of dysfunctional proteins)

- lowers the level of insulin in the blood;

- reduces the level of inflammatory processes;

- enhances antioxidant protection (if there is a lot of sugar in the diet, oxidative damage occurs, oxygen free radicals increase, which damage proteins, lipids, DNA and more);
- activates mitochondria;

- normalizes the level of stress hormones and appetite;

has a positive effect on neurotrophic factors in the brain (these molecules help the body to cope with stress, react to it in time and recover from it, it is low-carb and ketogenic diets that increase its level).

Disadvantages and benefits of fast diets:

- Minimal psychological stress.

- The shorter is the diet, the less stress the body is exposed to;

- Ease of compliance.

With fast weight loss, most often you do not need any special menu. Fast results. In a few days, you can lose from two to four kilograms.

But fast diets have their drawbacks:

- imbalance of elements and vitamins valuable for the body;

- decreased performance;

- there is a high probability of returning lost pounds immediately after the end of the diet;

- discomfort in the stomach at the end of the period of weight loss.

**Cleansing or detox diets**

According to statistics, in 60% of cases, the problem of slagging of the body can be solved with the help of special nutrition. There are foods that neutralize poisons and eliminate toxins.

Some products, on the contrary, promote the penetration of toxins into the intestines and blood, then they are carried through all systems.

Based on this, various options for cleansing diets are being developed - depending on what result you want to achieve or which organ needs a general cleaning.

**Mono-diets**

The essence of the mono-diet is that for several days the entire daily diet should consist of only one product.

The first and foremost advantage of any mono diet is fast weight loss in a short time. Mono-diets are effective, especially for quick weight loss. Depending on the chosen product, the duration of the mono-diet and the metabolic rate in the body, you can lose up to 4-5 kg in 3 days.

Mono-diets are also attracted by their ease of use: there is no need to invent special dishes and spend time preparing them, while a completely pleasant and even favorite product is chosen for eating. And a mono-diet will help to perfectly cleanse the body of toxins and excess fluid. A mono-diet for 1-3 days is an excellent unloading diet option that helps maintain a healthy body tone.

The main disadvantage of a mono-diet is that the body is under severe stress and at the end of the diet seeks to regain the lost pounds.

In addition, the use of a single product in a mono-diet can have harmful effects on the body.

According to nutritionists, the optimal period for observing any mono-diet is 7 days, and its maximum allowable duration is no more than 14 days.

Due to the severe restriction of the intake of nutrients into the body, a mono-diet can provoke dizziness, general weakness, distraction, headaches and decreased blood pressure. The mono-diet can be used with extreme caution in hypertension and diabetes; mono-diet is definitely prohibited during pregnancy, with urolithiasis, diseases of the gastrointestinal tract.

**Protein diets**

Protein diet, as the name implies, is based on the consumption of protein foods, while carbohydrate foods are minimized. Result: minus 5-10 kilograms in just ten days. By the way, that is how long it lasts.

Protein Weight Loss Diet is the perfect way to lose weight without suffering from constant hunger. This is possible due to the high protein content of the foods consumed.

- Ideal for athletes, as it allows you to maintain and build muscle definition in the process of getting rid of excess subcutaneous fat.

- There is no "saggy skin" effect.

- Along the way, it cleanses the body.

- Improves metabolic processes and speeds up metabolism.

- With the right approach and compliance with all the rules, it gives a sustainable result.
- Allows you to use a delicious and rich menu.

Disadvantages:

- Cannot be used for some diseases.
- 
- There is a leaching of calcium from the body.
- 
- The appearance of lethargy and weakness in the initial stages is possible.

# Preface

It seems that every day we learn about a new diet, we hear reviews about losing weight from friends, from the media or in social networks. Celebrities promote any diet, calling it - the only effective one. And then, we find that they eat differently.

Everyone wants to find a magic pill to lose weight. But we are all different. And what will fit your neighbor may not help you in any way. Stop blindly following ads or other people's opinions about diet. Create a nutritional strategy that will work for you! How to do it?

**Your ideal diet**

The diet that may guarantee to lose weight depends on your goals, activity level, type of your body, genetics and many other parameters. However, at the moment, many diets have a polar focus on food choices - low-carb, low-fat, high-protein, carnivore, vegan … Is it any surprise that so many people refuse diet as soon as they know what restrictions they will face!

People who have been successful in losing weight have tried or at least heard of many popular diets. However, they fully realized the futility of their attempts to follow the proposed nutrition plan at 100%. Their success began with a deep understanding of their body and what works only for themselves!

Is it diet - is our enemy! Or it's our  friend? Did you know that before the diet took on the meaning as a "limited menu for weight loss", it meant all foods consumed by humans? The thought of depriving yourself of your favorite food strains everyone at the molecular level.

Mice that were forced to go on a "diet" have shown elevated levels of stress hormones and instances of depressive behavior in rodents. Perhaps this is what induced mice to eat more junk food than on normal days without a diet ... Does this sound familiar?

Research the specifics of different diets, even if you have not yet chosen one that suits you.If you think about the details of any modern sufficiently researched diet, you can understand that they are not so different. Except for extreme diets, many popular diets such as paleo, low carb, high in protein, vegetable, etc. share several worthy values that anyone can follow.

The fact of choosing healthy products crowds out fast food and other unhealthy food. It's almost impossible to find a diet that actually encourages you to eat more unhealthy foods, this focus on your diet will ultimately lead to health and longevity.The diet can help control satiety and food intake.

Better quality foods usually lead to better digestion and metabolism, often because they contain fiber.

# Contents

Diet for the intestines

Porridge Diet

## Mono-diets

Rice Diet

Potato Diet

Orange Diet

Apple Diet

Soup Diet

Zucchini Diet

Choco Diet

Banana Diet

## Protein diets

Meat Diet

Prana Diet

Egg Diet

7 Petal Diet

# Fast Diets
## Diet "Weekly"

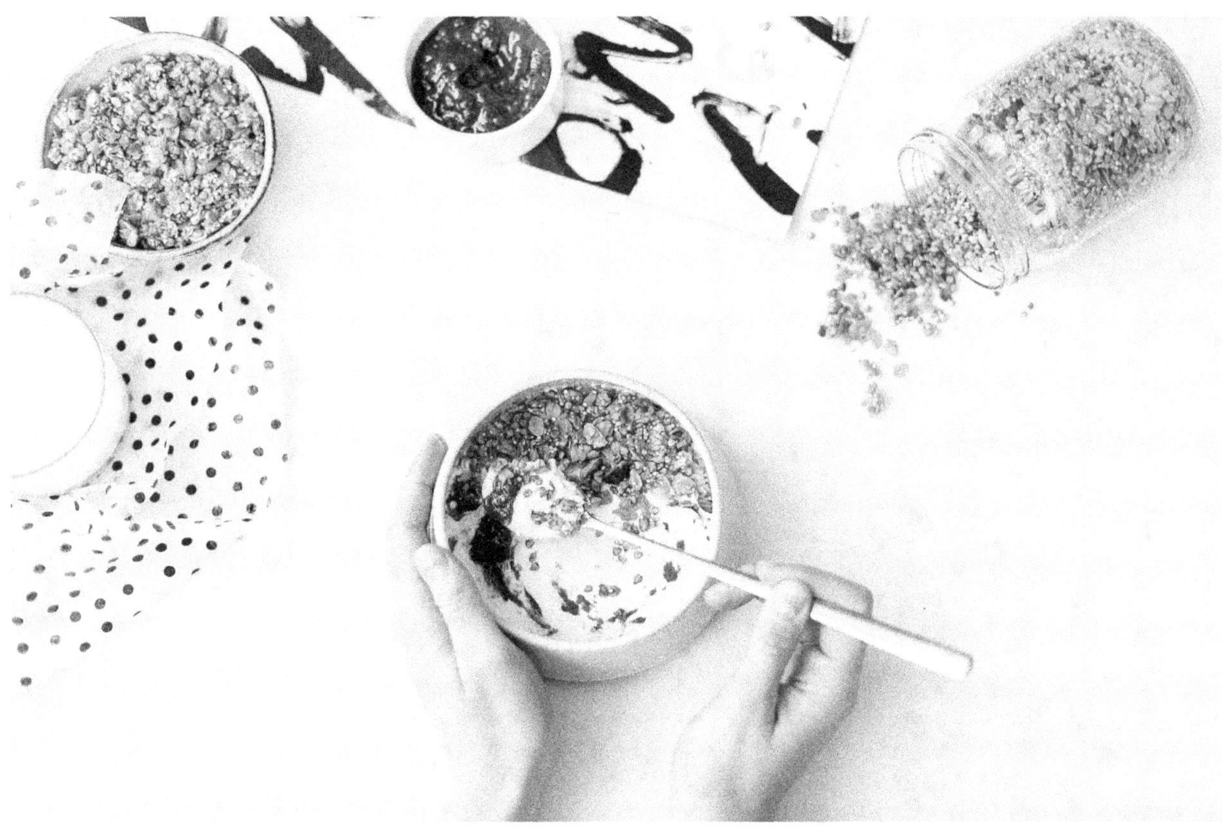

**Diet "Weekly" for effective weight loss**

This seven-day diet for weight loss refers to low-carb express methods. "Weekly" is difficult to comply, because it has "drinking days" (without food). Due to the low calorie content (less than the basic metabolism) and the imbalance of the diet, is considered rigid.

**The essence and effectiveness of the diet**

Getting rid of excess weight will help diet for weight loss in a week. It consists of 6 main days in which you need to eat fat-burning foods, and 1 transition - to return to your usual diet.

*According to nutritionists, the "Weekly" menu will not give the body the right amount of micro and macro elements, but the weight is leaving, so the system is considered effective.*

**The principles of the method of losing weight:**

- sharp decrease in caloric intake - up to 1000 kcal;
- alternation of protein and carbohydrate mono-diet with drinking days;
- strict adherence to the power scheme and menu.

For a week, according to reviews, you can lose 4-5 extra pounds and a few centimeters in the waist and hips. Achieving this result on a diet is due to the fact that:

- The body has to spend its own reserves of fat due to a lack of calories.
- Excess fluid is eliminated over 7 days and causes weight loss.
- Fiber from vegetables and fruits normalizes the intestines, which has a beneficial effect on the figure.

**"Weekly" Rules**

to lose weight on a 7-day diet, follow these rules:

1. 3-5 days before express weight loss, reduce the amount of high-calorie foods and serving volumes.
2. Eat 3 times a day without skipping meals.
3. Eat raw vegetables , cook the products without adding oil.
4. Follow the sequence of days of the diet and its menu: one product per day.
5. Drink up to 3 liters of clean water on "drinking days", and the rest of the time for 1.5–2 liters.
6. Exclude salt from the diet.
7. Exit the diet correctly so that lost kilos do not return. Gradually increase the daily amount of calories (by 100-150 kcal per day).
8. Use this system in the warmer months when you want more water than food, and the main menu products are fresh and available.

**Allowed foods**

The  7-day "Weekly" diet is based on the use of these foods:


- low-fat cottage cheese, fermented baked milk, yogurt and buttermilk;

- poultry (turkey fillet, chicken);

- meat (beef);

- vegetables (cucumbers, carrots, beets, tomatoes, zucchini, radishes, onions, broccoli, asparagus, bell pepper, olives);

- greens (arugula, salad, parsley, cilantro, celery, spinach, dill);

- eggs, buckwheat, olive oil;

- fruits (plum, melon, apple, mandarin, pomegranate, watermelon, pear, grapefruit, peach, pineapple, kiwi, nectarine and lemon);

- seafood, fish (flounder, cod, mackerel, pink salmon);

- berries (lingonberries, currants, blueberries, strawberries);

- dried fruit compote, green tea, vegetable juices, herbal decoctions and infusions.

**Partially or completely excluded products**

The "Weekly" diet also has a list of prohibited foods. Partly or completely excluded from the diet:

- sugar, salt;

- fatty meat (pork, lard, lamb);

- sausage products (sausages, sausages);

- oils (creamy, unrefined sunflower);

- beans, potatoes, peas;

- chips, crackers, fast food;

- smoked, fried, canned products;

- bananas, grapes;

- semolina, white rice, nuts, mushrooms;

- pasta, bakery, flour products;

- sweets, pastries, chocolate, honey;

- pickles, marinades, sauces, mayonnaise;

- alcohol, soft drinks, fruit drinks, fruit drinks, tea, coffee, energy.

## Week diet menu

This weight loss technique is suitable for people with good health. If there are chronic diseases, migraines, hormone problems - it is better to use the sparing version of the "Weekly". Unlike the main one, there are no drinking days and a balanced diet. The volume of products for each day of the week:

- 1st - 500 g lean meat;

- 2nd - 1.5 kg of vegetables, except for potatoes;

- 3rd - 5 chicken eggs (scrambled eggs, hard boiled);

- 4th — 750 g low-fat fish (steamed or baked);

- 5th - up to 1.5 kg of unsweetened fruits;

- 6th - 500 g fat-free cottage cheese or buttermilk;

- 7th - not more than 500 g of low-fat fish, meat; greenery.

The basic version of the "Weekly" is more strict.

### *Some recommendations:*

- Eat small meals 5-6 times a day.
- Drink boiled or still mineral water half an hour before meals or 40 minutes after it.
- On days when you are allowed to eat, only cook solid foods.
- Try to eat at the same time, dinner - until 19.00.

## The first "drinking day"

"Weekly" begins with the cleansing of the body, solid food is prohibited. Recommendations on the drinking scheme:

- clean water - 1.5–2 l in equal volumes (200 ml 7–10 times a day);
- permitted liquids - vegetable and fruit juices, unsweetened tea, herbal decoctions (1–1.5 l).

## Vegetable day of the "weekly" diet

At this time, it is allowed to eat any vegetables. Dietary recommendations:

- Use only permitted low-calorie foods.
- Eat raw vegetables individually or prepare a salad with lemon dressing or olive oil.
- Stew and bake some of the food if you can't eat raw food.

- Drink 2 liters of water.
- The last meal is 4 hours before bedtime.

## The third "drinking day"

The "Weekly" diet is distinguished by the alternation of hungry days (on water) with well-fed ones. On the third day, only fluids are consumed. If hunger overcomes, you can drink a glass of rice broth, low-fat chicken broth, natural yogurt, tea with milk.

## The fourth day -  fruits day

The body needs slow carbohydrates. They are found in sufficient amounts in unsweetened fruits. Recommendations on the menu of the fourth day of the Week:

- Eat an apple in the morning, it increases the feeling of hunger.
- Eat fruits in any quantities and variations - salads, slices.
- Add allowed berries to your diet.
- Try to eat more fat-burning fruits (citrus fruits, pomegranate, pineapple).
- Observe the water balance (2 l).

## Protein loading on the fifth day

After a fruit holiday in "Weekly" protein day is supposed. Nutritional recommendations:

- Eat fish, eggs, lean meat, low-fat cottage cheese.
- Steam food, bake without oil, boil without salt.
- Divide the daily amount of food into 5-6 servings of 100-150 g.
- Remember to drink plenty of fluids.

## Sixth day - water day

Diet with "drinking days" helps to reduce the volume of the figure. The sixth and last water day is easier to maintain than the first and third. If you use fruit juices, pay attention to calories and drink it immediately after preparation. But it is better to make juices from vegetables. Good to use smoothies, fresh, cocktails.

**Exit from the diet**

The last day of the Week is devoted to preparing for the transition to a normal diet.

Menu options:

- Breakfast - steam omelet from 2 eggs, apple (1 pc.), Green tea (150 ml).
- Snack - grapefruit (1/2 pcs.).
- Lunch - buckwheat soup (200 g), boiled turkey (100 g), broth of wild rose (150 ml).
- Snack - cottage cheese (150 g).
- Dinner - a salad of fresh vegetables with herbs and olive oil (200 g), buttermilk (150 ml).

**Advantages and disadvantages of the express diet**

Benefits of the "Weekly" diet:

- accessibility of the menu, especially in the season of fruits and vegetables;
- effective weight loss;
- eliminate the body from toxins;
- calories do not need to be counted;
- ease of preparation (most foods are consumed raw).

**The "Weekly diet" also has some disadvantages:**

- method of losing weight is contraindicated to pregnant and lactating women, children under 18 years old, people with diabetes, gastrointestinal diseases, oncology, metabolic disorders, and increased physical exertion;
- the diet is not balanced in micronutrient content;
- side effects - poor health, irritability, weakness, fatigue;
- hormonal disorders may occur;
- there is a risk of breakdown due to severe restrictions;
- gone kilograms can quickly return;
- You can't use the diet often (more than 2 times per year).

# Interval diet

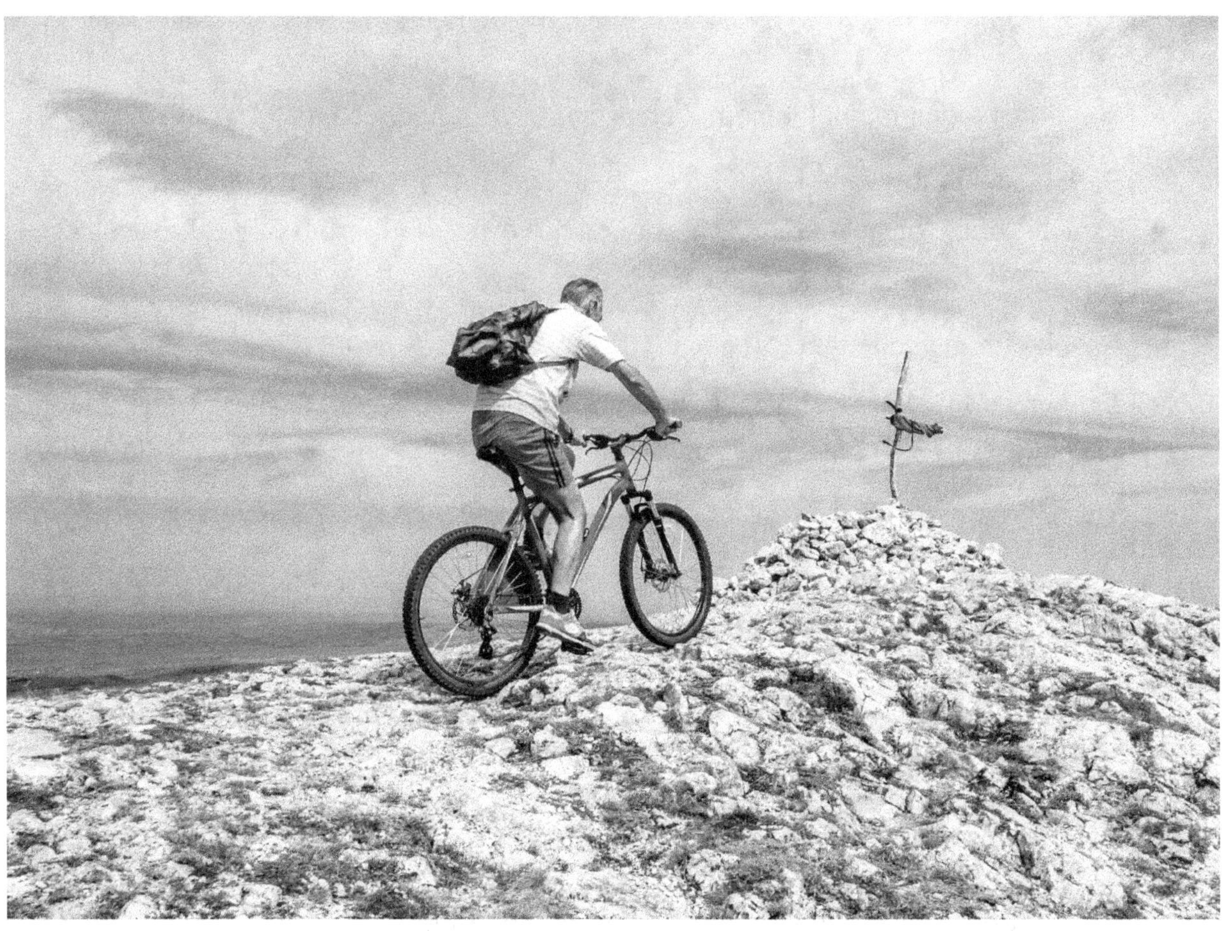

## Interval diet for weight loss by day

The essence of cyclic nutrition is that in a certain short period of time do not eat any food. This mode is practically independent of the list of allowed or prohibited products, and is based on when it is possible and impossible to take food. Periods of eating are replaced by intervals of abstinence from food.

## Principles

Intermittent Fasting is a cyclical diet without counting calories or irritability due to malnutrition. The fasting phase is slightly longer than the period of eating food.

*When the body digests food and no longer receives food temporarily, the burning of extra pounds begins.*

**Principles of Interval Nutrition:**

1.  The food window is designed to consume a daily calorie intake. Food can be fractional (5-6 times) or standard (3 large meals).
2.  During interval fasting, it is allowed to drink water, non-nutritious drinks (black or green tea, coffee without additives).

## Nutritional schemes for the resonance diet

With an interval diet, the day is divided into two periods, displayed in numbers that are indicated by a fraction: the "food window" and fasting. The effectiveness of different modes differs in degree of complexity and rate of decrease in body weight. Gentle fasting every other day, when unloading involves consuming about 500 calories - a very simple method to quickly and easily bring your body into shape.

There are more strict interval nutrition schemes that are not suitable for everyone, but only for people with good health who do not have chronic diseases. The interval diet is selected according to the initial body weight, gender, age, physical activity and other individual factors.

## Easy regimen of periodic fasting 12/12

This scheme of an interval diet is suitable for beginners or people who adhere to a fractional diet. Such an interval diet is observed, if necessary, at least for a lifetime. A 24-hour day is divided in half. For eating, 12 hours are allotted, for fasting - a similar time. There is also a complicated version of cyclic nutrition - 14/10. The periodic diet is easy to cope - at least 12 or 14 hours must elapse between dinner and breakfast.

This is a complex scheme of interval nutrition - the food window is only 8 hours, the rest of the day refrains from eating. In the phase when you can eat, it is allowed to eat any food and the prescribed amount of calories. An effective periodic fasting of 16/8 ensures fast weight loss with minimal energy consumption.

This interval diet scheme is suitable for long-term compliance (3-4 weeks) for both men and women, including those involved in sports. The optimal scheme of interval nutrition, in which there is a "drying" of the body.

*The effectiveness of a periodic diet is easy to increase, if you exclude from the diet of semi-finished products and other harmful products.*

## Diet for 3 days according to the scheme 20/4

This interval type of food means that the "food window" is only 4 hours, the remaining 20 is a period of hunger. The founder of this Spartan eating regimen is artist Ori Hofmekler. A strict three-day diet for weight loss allows you to get rid of 500-700 grams of excess weight per day, and with physical activity - up to 1 kg.

In the phase of hunger it is allowed to drink fresh vegetable or fruit juices, in addition to water, tea or coffee. It is allowed to have a snack with nuts, after a workout you can drink a glass of buttermilk, yogurt or eat 2 hard-boiled chicken eggs. In the four-hour period of the food window, it is allowed to consume everything except harmful products. The main thing is to keep order: first fiber, then proteins and fats, then carbohydrates.

## Intermittent fasting in 2/5 mode

An interval diet from Michael Mosley involves consuming a limited amount of calories in two days: men - 600 kcal in 24 hours, women - 500 kcal. The remaining five days are the usual diet with a standard calorie intake corresponding to gender, body weight, lifestyle, and body characteristics. This intermittent feeding regimen is suitable for prolonged use until the desired body weight mark is reached (approximately 1 to 3 months).

## Advantages and disadvantages of cyclic fasting

Interval diet helps to dry the body and "draw" the muscle corset, therefore it's widely used in bodybuilding. The main thing is that training should be performed at the end of the phase of hunger, then fat is burned faster.

## Advantages of a interval diet:

1. Do not have to change your usual diet.
2. Neither calorie counting nor diet containers are required.
3. The level of the hormone ghrelin, which controls appetite, is normalized.
4. There is rapid weight loss, accelerated metabolism.
5. Excess fat is broken down, not muscle.
6. The production of growth hormone increases, which contributes to the renewal of body tissues and rejuvenation.
7. Phagocytes (cells of the immune system) are activated, which contributes to the healing of various diseases.
8. The gastrointestinal tract and liver are eliminate the toxins.
9. The level of "bad" cholesterol is reduced about 30%.

According to experts in the field of proper nutrition, an interval diet with long breaks in food is detrimental to health. Long intervals between meals slow down metabolic processes. A decrease of glucose during the period of abstinence from eating foods, when food enters the body again negatively affects the brain. Other disadvantages of the interval diet is:

1. Correction of the diet can not be avoided: the basis of nutrition should be natural, unprocessed foods, mainly proteins and complex carbohydrates.
2. Nutritional deficiencies can develop due to malnutrition.
3. Too much roughage rich in fiber can cause gastritis.
4. A prolonged change in diet adversely affects the menstrual cycle.
5. It will take you to get used to long breaks in food, at first breakdowns, expressed in overeating, are possible.
6. Interval hunger strikes cannot be observed for a long time, since a well-functioning digestion process is disrupted.
7. There is a risk of kidney stones or gall bladder formation.

## Interval diet results

Cyclic fasting is a viable and effective strategy for weight loss.

*Depending on the selected interval feeding scheme, it is possible to achieve burning from 1.5 to 3 kilograms of excess weight on a three-day system of 20/4 or 16/8.*

A longer diet for 9 days will allow you to get a result minus 5-10 kg.

If you adhere to the gentle schemes of periodic fasting 12/12, 14/10, 2/5, then losing weight will be slow, but systematic, from 3-5 kilograms per month or more. According to reviews of women who have tested the interval type of food, for 3 weeks you can lose 6-7 kg without exhausting hunger strikes. Athletes and those who visit the gym achieve similar results in 7-10 days.

According to ongoing research in the field of human nutrition and physiology, some fasting - will benefit the body. It is an evolutionary feature of homosapiens. In the absence of supermarkets and refrigerators, people calmly went without food for most of the day, while obesity was not as common as in the 21st century.

**Contraindications**

Interval nutrition is forbidden to practice for people with a body mass index below 17, as well as for patients with bulimia, anorexia and other eating disorders. Women with menstrual disorders are not recommended to limit their diet. Other contraindications for the interval diet:

- pregnancy and lactation;
- pathology of the cardiovascular system;
- age up to 18 years, when the body is in the stage of active growth;
- chronic gastrointestinal diseases (gastritis, peptic ulcer of the stomach and duodenum);
- liver problems
- carbohydrate metabolism disorders, diabetes mellitus.

# Diet "Deuce"

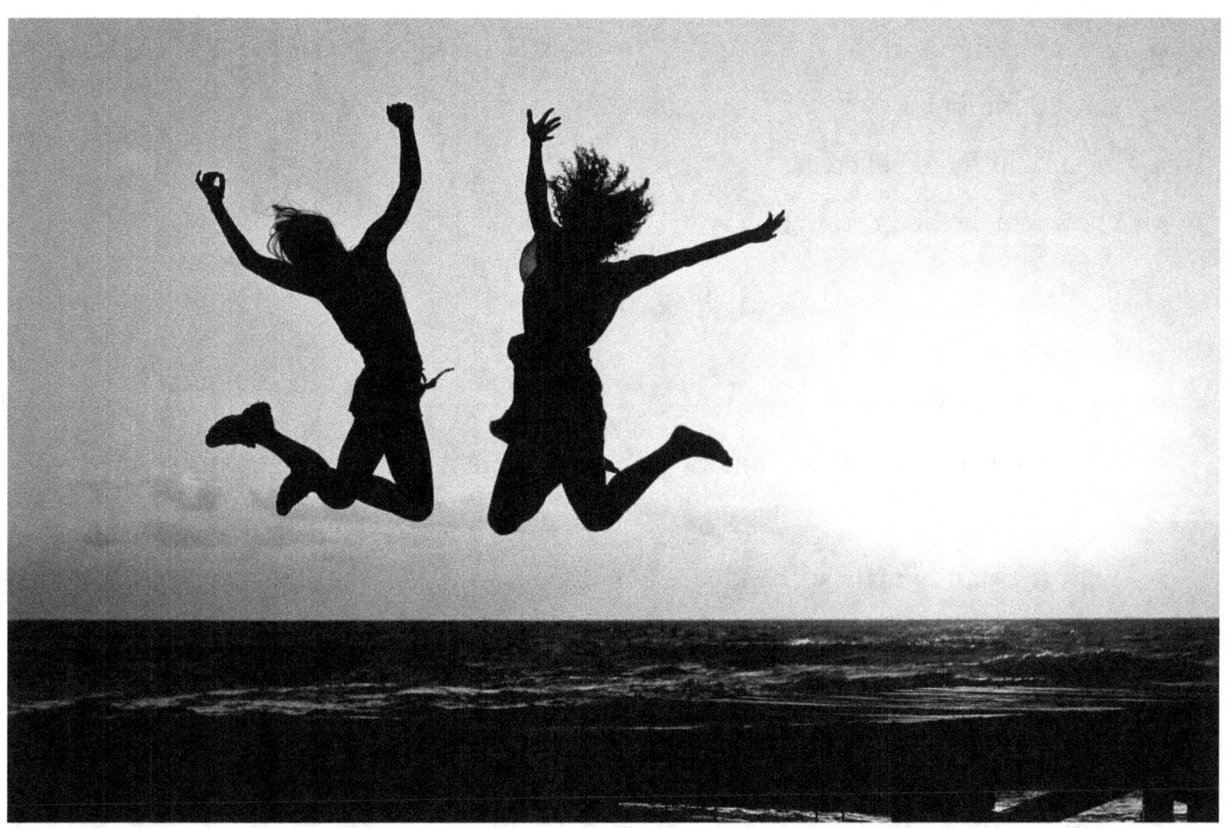

**Diet Deuce for weight loss by day**

The essence of the method of losing weight is the daily use of 2 units of food, 200 grams of food or 2 liters of liquid. Duration of the diet - no more than 10 days. During this time, it will take from 5 to 8 kg, depending on the initial weight. This result is achieved due to strict observance of the menu, preparation of the body for the diet and the rules for getting out of it.

**Advantages and disadvantages of the diet Deuce**

The main advantage of such a diet is rapid weight loss.

*Lack of calories "makes" the body go into stress mode and break down its own fat reserves.*

**Other advantages of the "Deuce":**

- high efficiency;
- guaranteed result;
- short duration;
- minimum financial costs;
- eliminate the body from toxins;

**Disadvantages of the "Deuce":**

- rigid diet causes stress;
- due to a lack of vitamins, minerals, fragility of nails, hair, and peeling of the skin may occur;
- with starvation, malaise, headaches, nausea, powerlessness, lethargy, pressure surges, half-fainting conditions are possible;
- 3-4 days, you may smell acetone from the mouth.

## Preparing for a diet

The "Deuce" nutrition is limited, this is a low-calorie diet. In order for the body to experience less stress during weight loss, it needs to be ready. It may done in 3 stages:

1. Smooth transition to proper nutrition. 2 weeks before the diet, gradually eliminate harmful foods from the diet: pickles, smoked meats, sweets, flour, confectionery, fried and greasy foods, and carbonated sugary drinks. Refuse salt, spices, seasonings. Make a list of high-calorie foods and cross out 1-2 points daily.
2. Reduced daily calorie intake. Keep a food diary, write down everything you eat there in a day and count calories. Every day, reduce the number of kilocalories by 100-200 units. A week before the start of the diet, daily calorie intake should be no more than 1200 kcal.
3. Preparing for the famine. The essence of this stage is the rejection of solid food. So the body will well accept the limited low-calorie diet. On the first day, take the last meal no later than 18 hours, the second - until 16, the third - until 14, the fourth - until 12, on the fifth - only have breakfast. Sixth day - drinking. Allowed broths (without salt), low-fat dairy and sour-milk products without additives, unsweetened tea, coffee, cocoa.

**The basic rules of diet food**

Slimming with the "Deuce" gives a good result - the plumb will be 5-8 kg in 10 days. You can achieve it by observing certain rules:

1. Before starting to lose weight, cleanse the intestines with an enema adding chamomile, motherwort (2 tbsp. In 200 ml of water) or a saline laxative (2 tbsp. of sea salt per 1 liter of water).
2. Drink at least 2 liters of table water or mineral water without gas daily.
3. Do not swap diet days and foods on the menu.
4. Try to eat at the same time.
5. Have dinner no later than 7-8 o'clock in the evening.
6. Follow the rules for exiting the "Deuce" diet.

**Menu for weight loss**

The proposed diet must be strictly observed. Follow the drinking regimen. In addition to water, unsweetened coffee without milk, tea with cinnamon and ginger powder are allowed. Ten-day diet menu:

1. 1st day: apple (unsweetened varieties) - 2 pcs.;
2. 2nd: citrus fruits (tangerines, oranges, grapefruit) - 2 pcs.;
3. 3rd: oatmeal on water or boiled rice (unpolished) without oil, salt - 100 g;
4. 4th: hard cheese throughout the day (200 g), 1 tbsp. buttermilk for the night;
5. 5th: cottage cheese with a low percentage of fat content (without sugar and other sweeteners) - 240 g;
6. 6th: banana (unripe, unsweetened) - 2 pcs.;
7. 7th: only water;
8. 8th: fresh cucumber, yogurt (natural, without additives) - 2 pcs.;
9. 9th and 10th days: buttermilk - 2 l.

**Exit "Deuce" diet**

During this diet, the volume of the stomach is reduced, the metabolism is slow down.

*A quick return to the previous diet will lead to the deposition of fat in the body "in reserve" and weight again.*

**The correct way out of the "Deuce" diet will help to avoid following:**

1. Increase the volume of servings gradually.
2. In the first week, do not launch fatty, spicy, salty foods into the diet. Try not to salt the dishes.
3. Eat more with fresh, boiled, baked or steamed foods.
4. Prefer low-fat dairy, sour-milk, meat and fish products.
5. Salads season with a little olive oil with lemon juice.
6. After 7 days, launch meat, vegetable broths, your favorite dishes into the diet. Make sure that the daily calorie value is increased daily by no more than 50–80 units. Gradually bring it to its previous level - 1800–2000 kcal.

**Contraindications:**

The diet "Deuce" has some contraindications. It restricted to lose weight :

- during menstruation;
- during pregnancy, lactation;
- in the presence of allergic reactions to menu products;
- with increased physical and mental stress;
- during stress;
- in the presence of chronic diseases of the internal organs;
- in the preoperative period;
- in case of sleep disturbance;
- with deterioration in well-being with the disease;
- when changing the time zone.

# GM Diet

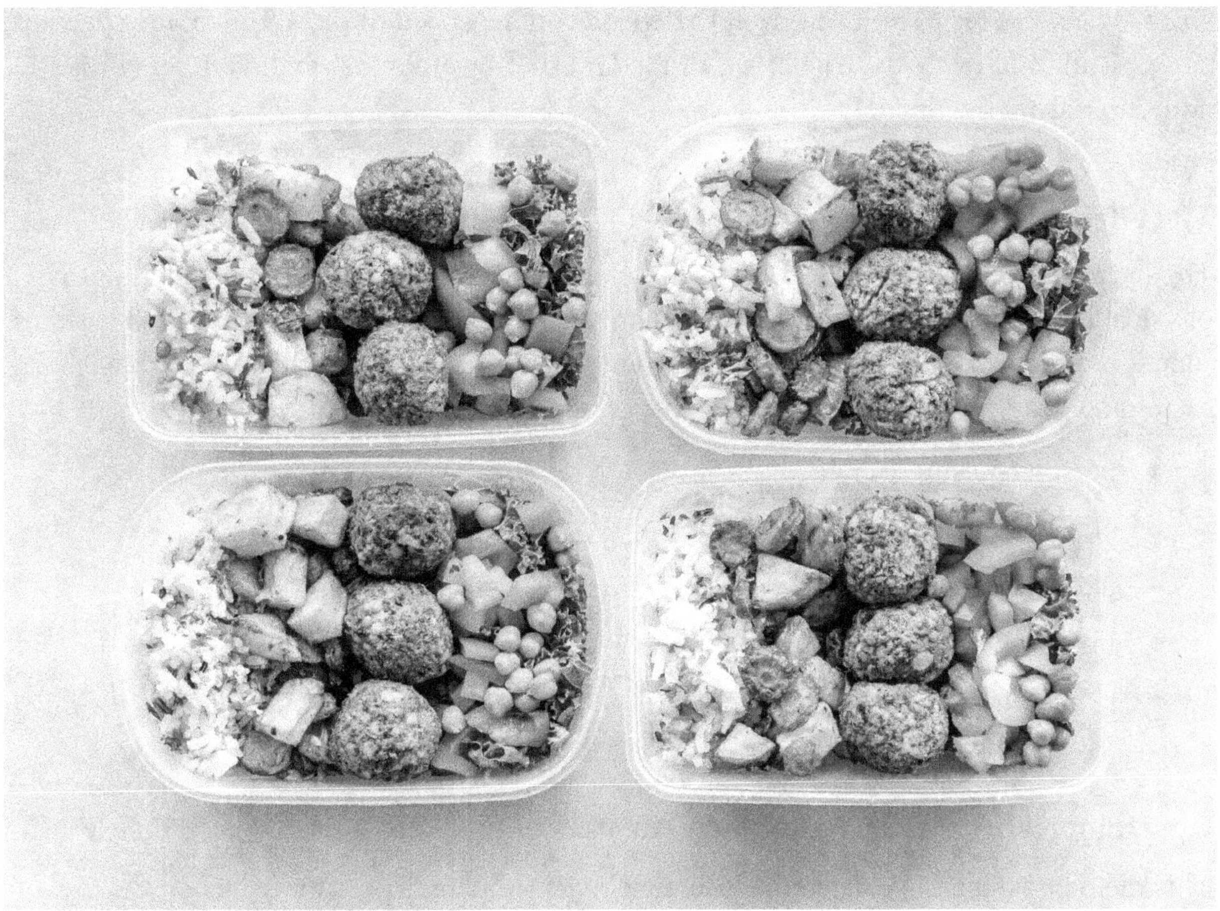

## General Motors Diet: Weekly Menu

A special diet was developed in the early 1980s by order of the US General Motors automobile concern. The owners of the largest company planned that the GM diet will improve the physical condition of employees, help increase productivity.

## The essence of the GM-diet

With GM diet, a person does not feel a debilitating hunger. The complex for weight loss and body healing is designed for 7 days. The weekly program is aimed to use allowed products from the list which is strictly regulated.  The diet includes fruit, vegetable, fruit and vegetable, banana-milk, protein days.

General Motors low-calorie diet affects not only body fat. The detoxification of the body occurs due to the receipt of a large amount of structured fluid, which is found in vegetables, fruits, and berries. It burns more calories than comes with food. Vitaminized foods contribute to increased physical activity.

## How much you can lose on a General Motors diet

Adhering to GM's wellness system, you can lose 3–7 kilograms of excess weight in a week. The rapid result of losing weight depends on the speed of metabolism, the speed of detoxification of the body. The effect of the GM diet - weight loss and well-being - is noticeable from the first days.

## The effect of diet on the body

The intake of vitamins, minerals, and trace elements in large quantities helps to improve physical activity. The body is freed from harmful substances, internal organs and systems function more actively. Increased labor productivity due to the fact that work is done easier and faster. After a week-long course on the GM diet:

- person is losing weight;
- eliminate the body from toxins;
- harmful cholesterol is excreted;
- immunity is strengthened;
- skin color, hair condition improve.

## Contraindications and possible side effects.

This diet is not suitable for people with digestive problems. Do not infringe on the diet of pregnant and lactating mothers. When the body is exhausted, it is also better to refrain from restrictions on food.

*To avoid side effects, you must follow the General Motors diet period - 7 days.*

Overuse can lead to vitamin deficiency. The low protein content and the almost complete absence of fat in the GM diet leads to the following pathologies:

- cognitive mental disorders (worsening of the process of memorization, irritability, depression);
- hormonal disorders
- decrease in the body's defenses.

## GM nutrition scheme:

Every day you need to drink at least 2 liters of water. There is no ban on green or herbal tea, natural coffee without additives.

*In the first 3 days, minimize physical activity due to possible weakness due to a change in diet.*

In the 2nd half of the week, physical exercises are useful, they contribute to the effective loss of extra pounds.

## Fruit day

On 1 day you need to eat any fruit, except bananas. Give preference to sweet and sour fruits or berries. All citrus fruits, kiwi, pineapple, green apples, strawberries, gooseberries, red or black currants have a fat burning effect. Approximate fruit and berry menu of the GM diet for 1 day:

- breakfast: several slices of watermelon or melon;
- 2 breakfast: green apple;
- lunch: 1-2 pears;
- afternoon snack: grapefruit;
- dinner: 3 kiwi;
- snack 2-3 hours before bedtime: seasonal berries or fruits.

## Vegetable

On this day, eat raw vegetables riching with fiber (white cabbage, broccoli, carrots) or dishes from it. The exception is starchy root crops (potatoes, Jerusalem artichoke and others). Make a salad, mashed potatoes or stew it. To improve the taste, you can add vegetable oil. On vegetable and fruit days, the portion size can be 300-400 g. An approximate menu of a vegetable day diet:

- breakfast: cherry tomatoes;
- 2 breakfast: salad of tomatoes and cucumbers with herbs;
- lunch: steamed cauliflower;
- afternoon snack: carrots;
- dinner: steam broccoli;
- snack: white cabbage salad with herbs.

**Fruit and Vegetable**

On the 3rd day of the GM diet, eat any vegetables and fruits except bananas and potatoes. Eat whole fruits or smoothies. They can be eaten fresh, steamed, boiled, stewed or baked. Sample menu of a fruit and vegetable day GM-diet:

- breakfast: apple;
- 2 breakfast: steam broccoli;
- lunch: a salad of fresh vegetables with herbs;
- afternoon snack: pomelo;
- dinner: avocado salad with cherry tomatoes, sweet pepper, arugula;
- snack: seasonal berries.

**Fruit and milk**

On this day, the diet consists of 6-8 bananas and 1 liter of milk, which are divided into 6 receptions. Bananas are a source of potassium and magnesium. These trace elements support the work of the heart. Milk enriches the body with calcium, phosphorus, and vitamin D.

**The final stage of the diet**

In 5–6 days, add 600 g of meat (mainly beef), poultry, or fish to the diet. Meat can be replaced with cottage cheese. Increase the water rate by 0.5 liters. On the 7th day of the GM diet, launch brown rice into the diet and eat vegetables, fruits, drink fresh juices in unlimited quantities.

**Recipes for the General Motors diet**

Vegetable soup or salad reduces hunger and helps remove excess fluid from the body. A few recipes for the General Motors diet:

**Dietary soup**

Ingredients:

- onions - 6 pieces (medium size);
- red pepper - 2 pcs.;
- tomatoes (large) - 4 pcs.;
- white cabbage - 1 pc. (small);
- celery - 1 bunch;
- any greens (dill, parsley) - 50 g.

Method of preparation:

1.  Pour 1 liter of water into the pan.

2.  Put chopped vegetables in boiling water.

3.  Cook for about 40 minutes.

4.  Season the soup with greens.

## Avocado Salad

Ingredients:

- Avocado - 1 pc.;
- cherry tomatoes - 5 pcs.;
- sweet pepper - 2 pcs. (red and orange);
- arugula - 20 g.

Cooking:

1.  Wash the vegetables.

2.  Peel the avocado and take out the stone.

3.  Pepper free from seeds.

4.  Chop all components, mix and add arugula.

## Vegetable salad with herbs

Ingredients:

- tomatoes - 2 pieces (medium);
- cucumber - 1 large or 2 medium;
- sweet pepper - 1 pc.;
- dill or parsley - 20 g.

Cooking:

1.  Cut the washed vegetables.

2.  Transfer to a salad onionl and mix.

3.  Sprinkle with chopped herbs.

# Anti-cellulite diet

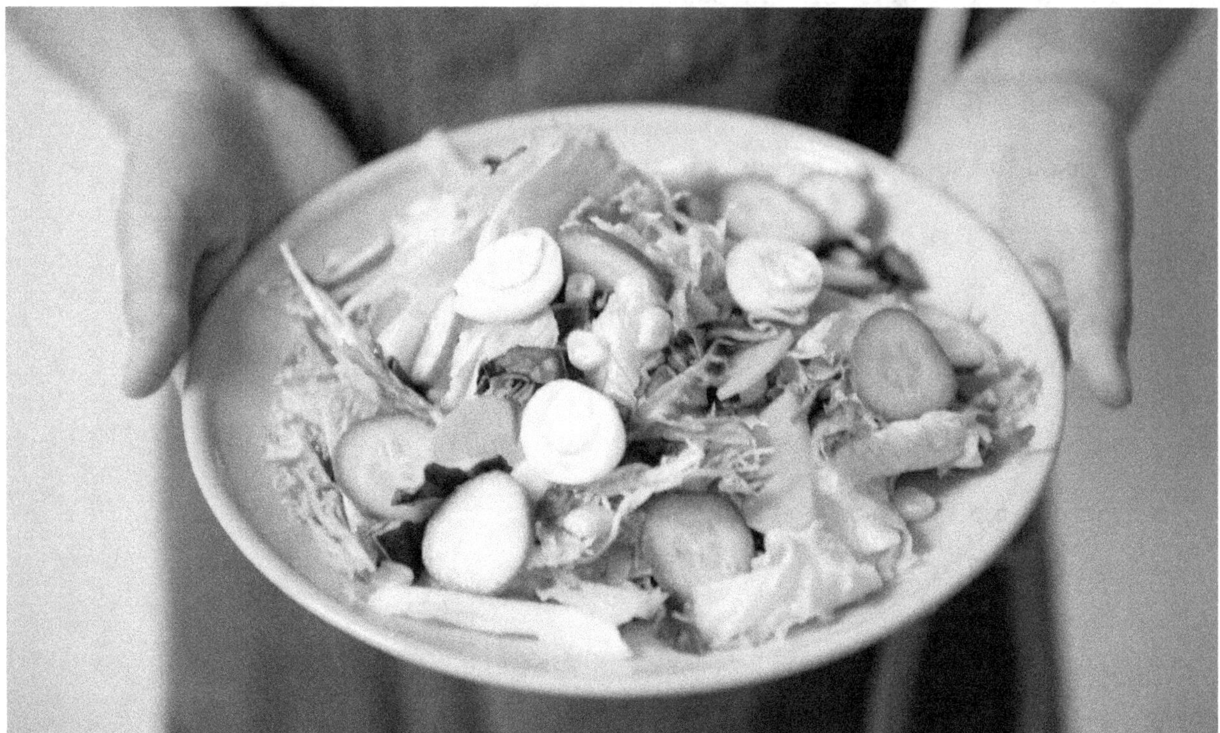

## Anti-cellulite diet nutrition

An extremely unpleasant, but very urgent problem for many women is cellulite. A special diet aimed at improving metabolism which will help to reduce cellulite availability. Anti-cellulite power system belongs to the category of hard. The diet is suitable for girls who want to get rid of the "orange peel."

## General Information about Cellulite

Many women, even those who maintain themselves in good physical shape, eventually find that the skin looks like an "orange peel". This phenomenon is called cellulitis - changes in the subcutaneous fat layer, accompanied by a violation of the microcirculation of the lymph flow. Women are significantly more prone to the problem than men. The main causes of cellulite and predisposing factors:

- unbalanced diet (the use of a large amount of carbohydrates, low - proteins and polyunsaturated fats);
- hereditary predisposition;
- constant fluctuations in weight;
- hormonal imbalance;
- violation of blood and lymph circulation in adipose tissue;
- non-observance of sleep patterns;

- violation of the water-salt balance, metabolism;
- frequent stresses;
- overweight;
- bad habits;
- lack of exercise.

**General rules of the anti-cellulite diet for 10 days**

The nutrition system eliminating the "orange peel" is aimed at improving metabolism, freeing the body of fats and waste substances. The diet of anti- cellulite is tough, but it helps to reduce its availability and lose weight by 3-4 kilograms in 10 days. Basic principles and rules of anti-cellulite nutrition:

1. Diet of anti- cellulite is based on the rejection of those products that contribute to fluid retention. It's strict dien and it belongs to the type of unloading

2. The main diet for 10 days of an anti-cellulite diet consists of fruits, vegetables, cereals from whole-zorn cereals. All of these products help improve onionel function. An anti-cellulite diet does not limit the serving size, but moderation is strongly recommended.

3. Salt, sugar, black tea, coffee should be categorically refused. Only vegetable oil remains in ration.

4. On days when boiled vegetables are allowed, 2 tbsp can be added of boiled cereals: brown rice, oatmeal, buckwheat or barley.

5. It is important to observe not only a diet with an anti-cellulite effect, but also a "drinking" regimen, because heavy drinking helps to eliminate toxins. A day you need to consume at least two liters of fluid.

6. With anti-cellulite nutrition, it is recommended to eat food every 2-4 hours in small portions.

7. Active sports for the period of diet should be abandoned in favor of calm walks.

**Healthy foods**

Vegetables and fruits are consumed fresh or in the form of salads in the anti-cellulite regimen. Anti-Cellulite products that are strongly recommended to be included:

1. Apricots, prunes, pineapple, strawberries. These fruits are rich in potassium.
2. Blueberries, grapefruit. Contains flavonoids, antioxidants. Good effect on the lymphatic system, strengthens blood vessels. Grapefruit has a substance called "naringin", which affects the secretion of insulin. Eating citrus fruits and blueberries will help suppress appetite, get rid of uncontrolled attacks of hunger, and burn body fat.
3. Avocado. Contains omega-3 acids, oleic acid. Promotes fat burning, suppresses appetite.
4. Pears Rich in iodine, which accelerates cellular metabolism.
5. White cabbage. It is rich in calcium, vitamin C, potassium.
6. Brussels sprouts. Contains diindolylmethane, which blocks estrogens that interfere with collagen synthesis.
7. Sprouts of soy, rye, beans, oats, corn, wheat, sesame seeds. Improve the taste of salads.


**Allowed**

Anti-cellulite diet for 10 days should be composed of vegetables and fruits, with a small addition of other products. What can definitely be eaten:

1. Vegetables, greens. Spinach, eggplant, lentils, celery, beans, beans, squash, pumpkin, all kinds of cabbage, tomatoes, cucumbers, asparagus, lettuce, soybeans, bell peppers, beets.
2. Fruits, berries. Black and red currants, avocados, grapes, oranges, apples, pomegranates, peaches, grapefruit, papaya, pears, nectarine, kiwi, lemons, tangerines, mangoes, watermelons, melons.
3. Dried fruits, nuts. Sunflower seeds, cashews, sesame seeds.
4. Cereals, cereals. Brown and brown rice, buckwheat, oatmeal.
5. Milk products. Natural yogurt 2% fat.
6. Seasonings. Sunflower and olive oils, dried herbs, honey.
7. Beverages. Mineral water, green tea.

**Prohibited**

Salt, sugar, alcohol anything that contains caffeine should be completely excluded from the diet.. In anti-cellulite mode, you can't eat fried, fish and meat can either be boiled or baked. Pasta made from wheat flour, white rice, pastries, canned goods, smoked meats, sausages fall under the prohibition of the diet. Pickles, pickled products also retain moisture in the body and stimulate appetite, so it needs to be excluded. The cheeses should be limited to the anti-cellulite regimen. List of banned foods:

- horseradish;
- salt;
- semolina;
- sugar;
- pasta;
- mayonnaise;
- wheat bread;
- mustard;
- jam;
- chocolate;
- jam;
- cakes
- potatoes;
- sweets;
- ice cream;
- biscuits;
- high fat milk;
- black tea;
- pork;
- coffee;
- sausages;
- smoked meats;
- canned food.

## Menu

It is known that the diet menu with anti-celulite effect is divided into even and odd days.On days 1,3,5,7,9 only fresh fruits and vegetables are permitted. Serving size is not limited, but try to control your appetite, do not eat too much. Example menu for an odd day diet:

| Eating | Diet |
| --- | --- |
| Breakfast | Allowed fruits in any quantity. |
| Lunch | A few pumpkin seeds. |
| Lunch | Fresh vegetable salad with olive oil. |
| Afternoon | Fruits |
| Dinner | Vegetable salad with sprouted wheat, oat, soy or bean sprouts. |

The whole second day of the diet, eat only fruits. You can take anything except bananas. Diet 4, 6 and 8 days of the diet - raw fruits and vegetables in any quantity, 2 tablespoons of cereals from the list of allowed, low-fat yogurt. Example of an even-day menu:

| Eating | Diet |
| --- | --- |
| Breakfast | Any fruit, a glass of freshly squeezed orange juice. |
| Lunch | 200 ml of natural yogurt. |
| Lunch | Spring salad with olive oil and equal in volume amount of vegetables boiled or stewed in water. |
| Snack | Salad from bell pepper, cucumbers, tomatoes, cabbage. |
| Dinner | 2 tbsp. l boiled buckwheat porridge, stewed vegetables, fruit salad (seasoned with yogurt). |

## Diet with anti-cellulite massage

To deal with the "orange peel" you need a comprehensive, only then you can achieve the result. A course of anti-cellulite massage in combination with a diet will be very effective. During its passage, you need to follow these nutrition rules:

1. Eat on a diet schedule. Five meals a day at regular intervals.
2. Reduce your intake of sugar and salt.
3. Exclude alcohol, convenience foods, fast food, flour, sweet, fatty and other junk food.
4. Follow the "drinking" regimen.
5. Make a diet of vegetables, fruits, foods high in protein and omega-3 acids, sprouted grains, whole grains. Nuts, avocados, seeds, low-fat fish, and seafood are

suitable.

6. From drinks is suitable mineral water without gas, freshly squeezed juices, green tea, herbal infusions, compotes.

## Exit from the diet

Following the usual mode - you need to smoothly, gradually expand the diet. So that cellulite does not form, you need to eat properly, and not the same as before. Thinking over your daily diet after the anti-cellulite diet has ended for 10 days and be guided by the following principles:

1. Daily calorie content - 1800 kcal. A prerequisite after a diet is to exercise three times a week.
2. Nutrition for cellulite should be frequent. Have three main meals and two snacks.
3. The basis of your diet should be fruits and vegetables, legumes, whole grain cereals and everything that is rich in potassium.
4. Use only vegetable oils.
5. Snacking after a diet, eat seeds, nuts. It has a lot of fiber, potassium and unsaturated fatty acids.
6. Even after the diet, reduce the usual amount of animal fats, salt, sugar consumed. Cheese can be eaten no more than three times a week and no more than 60 g per day.
7. Give preference to drinks such as decaffeinated coffee, fresh, green tea.
8. Replace sugar by honey.
9. Rare - it may be dairy products. Choose low-fat dairy products.
10. Refuse wheat bread in favor of bran, rye, whole grain and wholemeal.
11. Try to replace sweets with fruits and juices with pulp.

Although there are many restrictions, you can make a varied diet of the allowed foods. An example of a menu for two days of constant nutrition for women who are struggling with cellulite:

| Meal | 1 day | 2 day |
| --- | --- | --- |
| Breakfast | 2 tbsp.corn flakes, 1 tbsp. nuts, 1 tbsp. oat bran, 100 g of black currant, 150 ml of natural yogurt, a cup of green tea. | 1 slice of whole grain bread, 1 tbsp. peanut butter, 1 orange, a cup of green tea. |
| Lunch | 2 whole grain cookies, 1 orange. | 1 cereal bar, 1 large nectarine. |
| Dinner | 200 g of boiled chicken breast, 250 g of salad from boiled green beans, lettuce and half of bell pepper, a loaf of bran flour, a glass of tomato juice. | 200 g turkey roll with spinach, bran bread, 200 g boiled lentils and greens, 2 kiwi. |
| Snack | 150 g of natural yogurt. | 120 ml of skim milk, 100 g of muesli. |
| Dinner | 150 g of baked fish, 200 g of stewed vegetables (carrots, Brussels sprouts, celery, leek). | 120 g of baked halibut, 150 g of carrot and cabbage salad with sesame oil, 1 apple. |

# "Ladder" diet

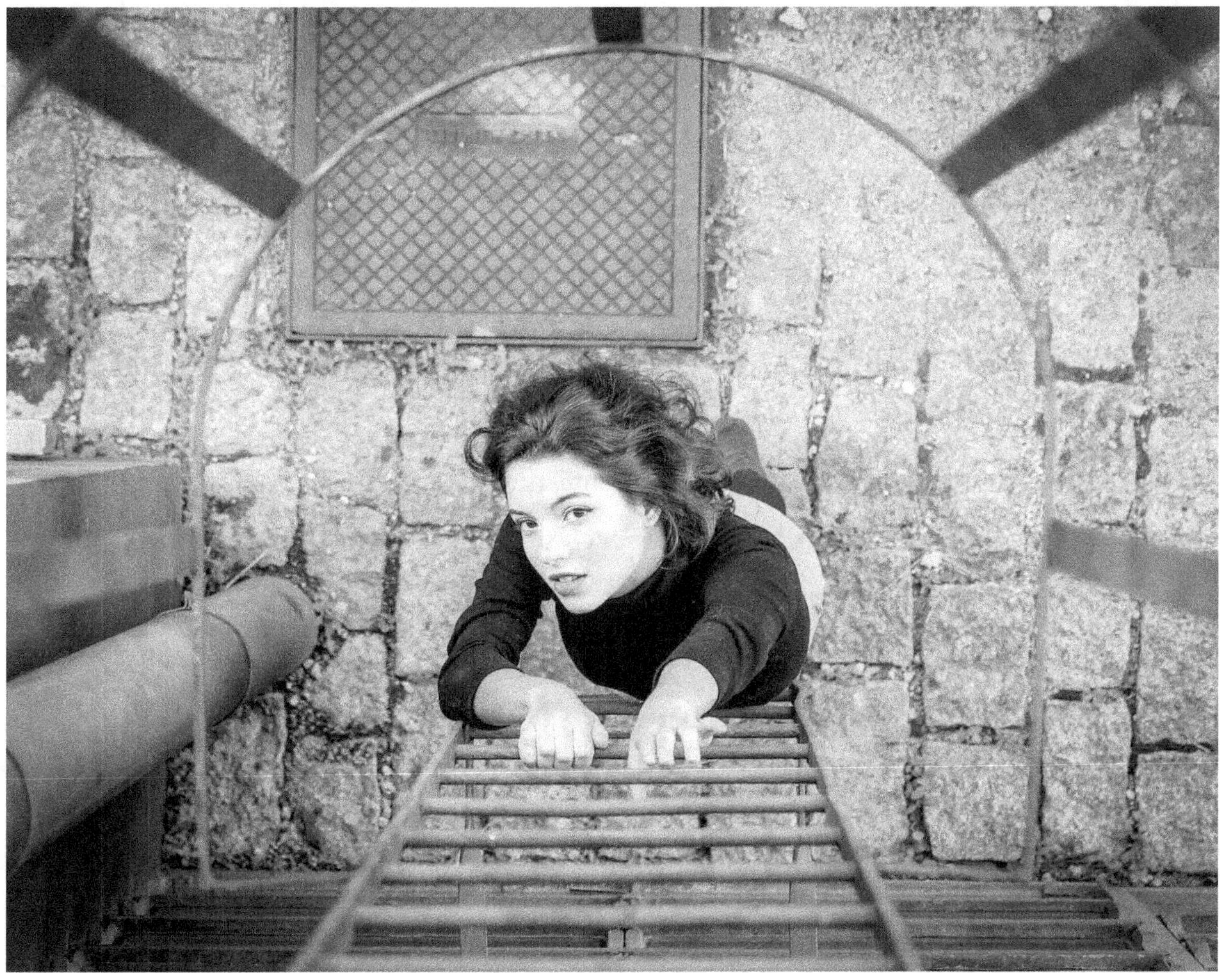

## Ladder diet: menu for 7 days

There are many different methods with which you can get rid of extra pounds. Some of them are designed for long-term, while others promise quick weight loss in a few weeks. Diet Ladder involves observing a limited diet for only 7 days. According to the reviews - it is possible to lose up to 8 kg.

## Rules and principles of the Ladder diet

The name of the diet scheme for weight loss is closely related to the diet idea: you have to go through 7 steps, sometimes not quite easy, to say goodbye to excess volumes of the waist, stomach and hips.

The Ladder Diet for 7 days refers to fast low-carb diets. Its basic principles are based on the use of a minimum amount of calories per day. The following points should be taken into account throughout the entire weight loss phase:

- diet is unbalanced, therefore, to replenish the supply of vitamins and minerals, start taking multivitamin complexes several days before it.

- every day you can eat only a certain type of food, while it is forbidden to eat in large portions. The menu needs to be designed so that snacks are every 2-3 hours.
- Be sure to drink plenty of fluids - up to 2 liters per day. Suitable mineral non-carbonated water, herbal tea, broth of wild rose, chicory.
- To maintain the beauty of hair and nails, you can take special biologically active additives .
- To achieve good results, you must clearly adhere to the menu. If you get lost or use a prohibited product - start over.
- The psychological attitude is no less important. Make sure you are ready for a weekly tight diet.
- To facilitate the process of losing weight - note, the results of each day, draw a ladder with 7 steps in a diary. Under each of them write the menu for the day, and at the end of the day enter your weight.
- Products that you abandoned while losing weight should be launched into the diet gradually no more than 2 per day.
- To get enough in small portions, nutritionists recommend chewing food slowly and concentrating.
- Diet Ladder does not exclude sports. If you feel good in the process of losing weight, do not forget about jogging, dancing, fitness or other physical activities.

**The menu of the five-stage diet for 7 days**

The Ladder slimming scheme is very convenient in that the menu of each day is clearly scheduled. Thanks to this, you don't have to think long about what products to make your diet from, how many calories are in beef or white bread. The basis of nutrition is made up of dairy products, turkey or other poultry, apples, honey, raisins and vegetables. Each type of product has its own purpose:

- Apples contain a large amount of pectin and perfectly satisfy the sense of hunger. Together with absorbents, it helps cleanse the intestines.
- buttermilk, yogurt, and low-fat cottage cheese contain live bifidobacteria - the basis of human microflora. Thanks to dairy products, you can avoid heaviness in the stomach, flatulence, constipation.
- Raisins with honey will help replenish the supply of energy spent, while the resulting supply of gluten will not be converted into fat by the body.

- Poultry meat will help not to break loose and manage the plan to the end, and will also contribute to the construction of muscle tissue.
- Vegetables are an excellent source of fiber, vitamins, and minerals. It will help consolidate the results achieved, relieve weakness and lack of nutrients.

The active phase of the Ladder diet falls on the first five days. For such a short period of moderate starvation, the body does not have time to go into a stressful stage, so the risk of side effects is minimal. Extending this diet for a longer period is strictly prohibited. The weight loss scheme is as follows:

- 1 stage - onionel cleansing;
- Stage 2 - normalization of microflora;
- Stage 3 - prevention of a breakdown, replenishment of energy deficit;
- Stage 4 - the formation of muscle tissue;
- 5th stage - fat burning;
- 6 and 7 steps - a smooth exit from the Ladder diet.

## Day 1 - Cleansing

At the first stage, preparing it for the process of losing weight,  it is necessary to cleanse the body from accumulated toxins. Pectin and a natural absorbent will accelerate metabolic processes, remove toxins, poisons and gases from the intestines. If you wish, you can replace black activated carbon with white, but keep in mind that its effectiveness is considered lower. The menu of the first day of the Ladder diet:

- 1 kilogram of green apples, which must be distributed throughout the day. Make sure that the meal is in regular intervals - 2-3 hours.
- 1-2 tablets of activated charcoal per hour before meals. In order for the absorbent to be better absorbed by the body, it must be washed down with plenty of water.
- One and a half to two liters of still or filtered water. Drink as necessary so that the body constantly replenishes the supply of fluid.

At the first stage, weight loss is about two kilograms, you should not stop there. The remaining steps are aimed directly at preparing the body and fat burning. Please note that on the first day, any food products are completely excluded, except for permitted, including tea, coffee or other drinks. Some women note that diarrhea occurs during the cleansing process. You should not be afraid of this symptom, the phenomenon will pass on its own, as soon as you move to the next step.

It is possible to facilitate the passage of the first day of the Ladder diet if you eat not fresh, but baked apples. The recipe for their cooking is simple:

1.  Thoroughly wash a serving of apples, cut in half and remove the core.
2.  Using a toothpick or fork, pierce the skin in several places so that the apples do not become cracked during cooking.
3.  Pour in a glass form for a microwave oven 2 tbsp. of water, put halves of fruit.
4.  Sprinkle apples with cinnamon if desired.
5.  Bake in the microwave for 5-7 minutes.

## Day 2 - Recovery

Having completely cleared the intestines of harmful substances in the first day, care should be taken to restore its microflora and work on the correction of digestive processes. Water, cottage cheese and buttermilk will help to cope with the tasks. Sour-milk products not only inhabit the intestines with useful bifidobacteria, but also saturate the body with protein, it helps to avoid weakness, dizziness and other unpleasant symptoms of starvation.

The approximate menu of the Ladder diet for the recovery period should look like this:

- After waking up, drink a glass of still mineral water. Eat 100 grams of cottage cheese of 0% fat mixed with a pinch of vanillin, mint leaves or cinnamon.
- For lunch, drink a glass of low-fat buttermilk. If desired, it can be replaced with yogurt or fermented baked milk with low fat content. Eat 100 grams of cottage cheese with mint.
- For lunch, take the same set of foods as for lunch. Mint in this case can be replaced with cinnamon. Drink a glass of water.
- Two hours after dinner, eat 70 grams of cottage cheese with vanilla, drink 200 ml of mineral water.
- The menu for dinner is similar to lunch, but at the same time you can mix the cottage cheese with buttermilk together. Remember that the last meal should be no later than 3 hours before bedtime.

**Day 3 - Energy**

After the first two days, the body will begin to experience energy malaise - weakness, dizziness will appear. This is due to the fact that during the first two stages almost the entire supply of glycogen, a polysaccharide, was spent, without which further weight loss would be very difficult. To replenish the supply of matter without depositing excess fat, you need to eat:

per day

- 400 grams of raisins;
- 2-3 tbsp. honey, divided into 4 doses;
- 2 liters of dried fruit compote.

Such a construction of the third day menu of the Ladder diet helps to avoid the effect of a plateau (weight fading). These products contain glucose, which will provide you with energy, but at the same time it will not increase the amount of subcutaneous fat. The stewed fruit will saturate the body with the necessary macronutrients: potassium, magnesium, iron. It is not difficult to prepare a flavored drink:

Soak 400 grams of dried apricots, 200 grams of dried apples or pears in warm water. Let the fruit swell a little.

1. Drain and add one and a half liters of clean liquid to the pan with dried fruits.
2. Put the container on the fire and cook for 20-30 minutes. If desired, before cooking, in a stewed fruit, you can add a carnation, lemon zest, 1 tbsp. apple syrup.
3. Allow the finished drink to brew for 2-3 hours, then strain.

**Day 4 - Construction**

Relative to the previous steps of the Ladder, the fourth stage will seem very high-calorie, satisfying and saturated. The goal of this day, as well as the previous one, is to prevent weight fading, but already with the help of protein products. The construction step helps to restore the supply of amino acids lost during the cleansing and restoration phase, improves the blood formation process and builds a muscle tissue. In the absence of discomfort at this point, you can enhance weight loss with exercise.

4 day involves eating white poultry. Suitable skinless chicken, turkey breast. All day you need to eat up to 0.5 kg of poultry and drink about one and a half liters of water. You can cook meat in any way - stew, fry without oil and salt. The turkey breast is very tasty if baked in an oven with herbs:

1. Preheat the oven to 180 ° C.

2. Brush the chicken breast with Dijon mustard (take about 300 grams) mixed with 50 ml of lemon and the same amount of soy sauce.

3. Leave the meat to marinate for 2 hours.

4. Put the fragrant breast on a baking sheet covered with foil. Sprinkle the meat with chopped caraway seeds on top.

5. Bake without closing the foil for 40 minutes.

## Day 5 - Fat Burning

The last stage of the Ladder is aimed at burning subcutaneous fat. The process of losing weight on the fifth day is due to use of low-calorie foods (bran, oatmeal, berries, fruits, vegetables) and the large expenditures of body energy aimed at digesting dietary fiber. The daily menu of the final stage looks like this:

- 300 g of oatmeal (weight of the product in raw form);
- 1 kg of any raw vegetables or fruits (with the exception of bananas, potatoes, peas, radishes);
- 1-2 liters of water without gas.

Oatmeal can simply be poured with boiling water in the evening or cook porridge from cereal in water without sugar and oil. The dish will turn out tastier if you add fresh berries and unsweetened fruits to it. Vegetables can be consumed separately or in the form of salads. To prepare a healthy snack you will need:

- white cabbage - 300 g;
- bell peppers - 2 pcs.;
- cucumber - 2 pcs.;
- parsley, dill or other herbs, spinach - to taste;
- vinegar - 1 tsp;
- olive oil - 2 tbsp.

## Cooking process:

1. Peel the cabbage from the top leaves and chop finely. Knead well with your hands.

2. From the peppers, remove the middle part and the stalk, cut into thin strips.

3. Cucumbers cut into circles or half rings.

4. Mix vinegar with olive oil.

5. Stir vegetables, add finely chopped greens.

6. Pour in the dressing.

## Day 6-7 - Exit from the diet

The goal of the last step of the Ladder is to consolidate the result and gradually return to the correct diet. The menu on the 6th and 7th day is not as sparse as the previous day. It is recommended to eat carbohydrates for breakfast, and protein for lunch and dinner. Servings should be small so as not to overload a fragile stomach, and frequent meals - 4-5 times a day.

Rice porridge with fruits boiled in milk with water helps to replenish the supply of energy, vitamins and amino acids. For 4 servings you will need these products:

- round-grain rice - 1 tbsp .;
- water - 2 tbsp .;
- sugar - 3 tbsp. .;
- milk - 1 tbsp .;
- salt - a pinch;
- any fruits or berries.

## Cooking process:

1. Rinse the rice under running water.
2. Boil water, pour prepared rice into a pan.
3. Reduce heat and simmer, stirring occasionally, for 10 minutes.
4. Pour sugar, salt, pour milk. Cook another 5-7 minutes.
5. Cover the finished porridge with a lid, decorate with fruit before serving.

In the middle of the day, it is important to eat a liquid dish - cream soup, vegetarian soup, chicken broth with dumplings. Well normalizes the digestive system pumpkin soup. It can be used:

- pumpkin - 750 g;
- carrots - 5 pcs.;
- onion - 3 pcs.;
- broth - 1.5 l;
- boiled chicken fillet - 200 g;
- greenery.

## The process of making pumpkin soup:

1. Cut the pumpkin into small pieces, fill with water, salt
2. Cook the vegetables

3. Grate carrots and onions with large holes. Passer in butter until golden brown.

4. Add the fried vegetables to the pumpkin, cook until cooked (40-60 minutes).

5. At the end, add chopped chicken breast and greens to the broth.

## What to do in case of a breakdown

The most difficult stages of the Ladder diet are unloading or purification and restoration. Many women endure the meager diet ration of the first two days, allowing themselves more than prescribed on the menu. According to the rules of the diet, this behavior is unacceptable. If you break down and violate a strict diet, you should interrupt the diet, pull yourself together and continue losing weight according to the scheme after 2-4 days.

## Contraindications

A sharp transition from a normal diet to a limited diet does not always benefit the body. Refuse from such a method of losing weight is necessary for those who have the following contraindications:

- inflammatory diseases of the gastrointestinal tract (gastrointestinal tract);
- liver, kidney disease;
- diseases of the cardiovascular system;
- oncological neoplasms;
- pregnancy;
- lactation;
- diabetes;
- hemorrhoids.

## Pros and cons of the Ladder diet

Due to a sharp change in diet, step-by-step diet of the Ladder can lead to intestinal upset - constipation, diarrhea, bloating. In addition, the results achieved on this weight loss scheme will not be long-lasting if after the completion, you fully return to your usual rhythm of life and menu. These significant disadvantages do not overlap the many positive aspects of the diet.

**Advantages include:**

- Easy tolerance. Many women note that adhering to the rules of the Ladder is much easier for them than aspects of other express diets. The main thing is not to go beyond the permitted products and drink the right amount of water.
- Availability of diet relative to the cost of products. All the dishes that are on the menu are inexpensive in the store, which makes Ladder even more attractive for many ladies.
- Simplicity. Serving sizes and allowed foods are strictly indicated in the diet. There is no need to count calories or figure out what to cook for tomorrow.

# Top Models diet

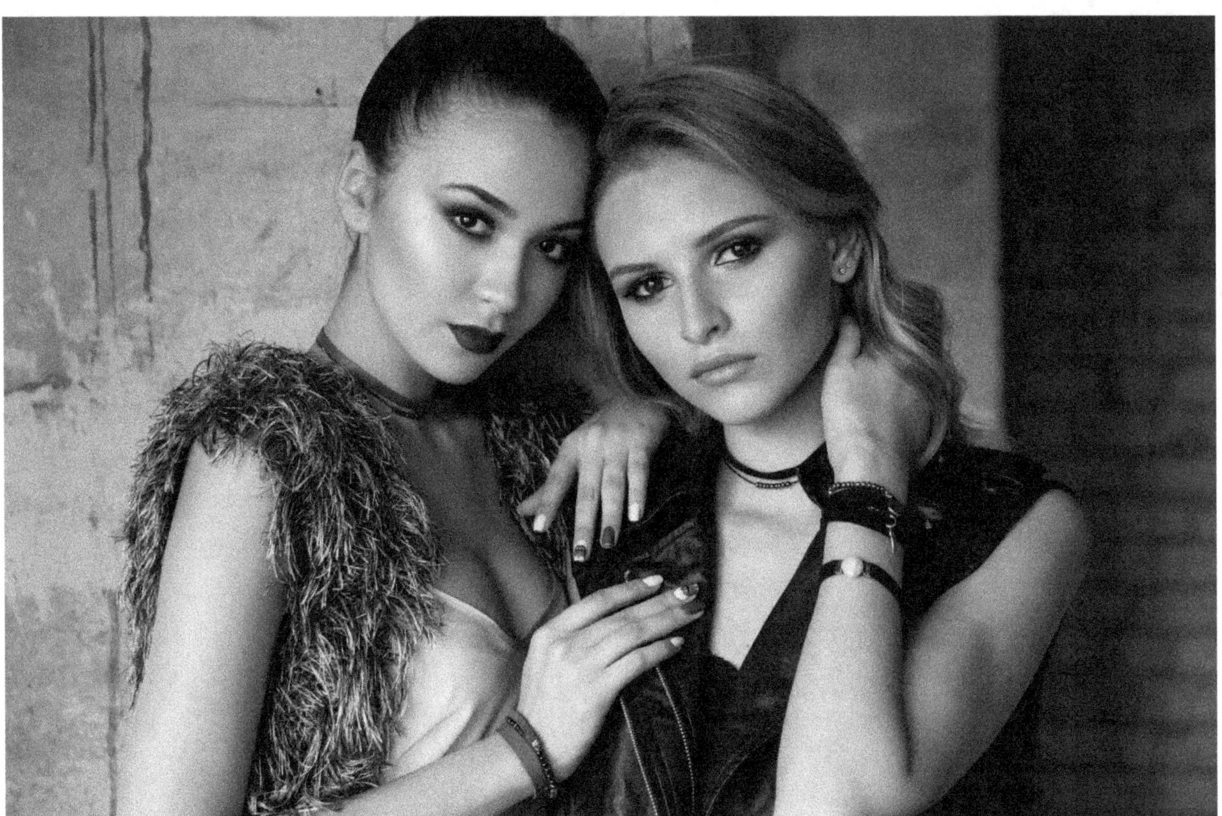

**Top Models diet for 3 and 7 days.**

Each model at least once in a life had to resort to emergency figure correction before casting.

**What is a top model diet?**

The body of the model is its working tool for demonstrating outfits or posing in front of cameras. In the modeling business, there are strict beauty parameters. When concluding a cooperation agreement, the model agrees to adhere to certain standards of appearance, which includes a body weight and volume.

Low-calorie models diet is designed for 3–7 days. During this time, it is realistic to lose 2.7 to 8 kilograms of excess weight. A strict three-day diet involves meals in the morning, and the weekly regimen is based on adhering to the schedule and reducing the amount of servings. The essence of the model's diet is to consume no more than 1000 calories per day. Weight loss is based on the use of low-calorie foods, compliance with the drinking regime, physical exercises, preferably in the fresh air.

A strict diet is suitable for everyone who wants quickly to get rid of extra pounds. In urgent cases at vacation or an important event is unexpectedly planned and it needs to look stunning, models' diets will help out. Diet restriction is contraindicated for persons with digestive system diseases or for individual indicators.

**The rules of the diet**

There is a lot of effort behind the perfect looks of top models or fashion models. Irregular work schedule, exhausting shows, hours of photo sessions, the use of tons of cosmetics on the face, body, hair - all this does not have the best effect on the appearance. Snacks, lack of sleep, fluid restriction 12 hours before the show lead to digestive problems, weight gain. Quickly bring the body back to normal will help a short-term diet for models, which has the following rules:

1. Breakfast is the main meal, never forget about.
2. Eat often, but in small portions. Fractional nutrition does not overload the digestive system.
3. Consume complex carbohydrates, completely eliminate simple carbohydrates.
4. Eat protein and carbohydrate foods at different times.
5. Avoid heavy loads. Do gymnastics and light training (yoga, Pilates, dancing).
6. Get fewer calories than you spend. Move as much as possible.
7. Follow the drinking regimen. Drink at least 1.7 liters of pure water per day. Drinking should be without additives, herbal tea is allowed.
8. Don't drink while eating. Drink half an hour before meals or 60 minutes after a meal.
9. Do not eat sweets and pastries, replace confectionery with dried fruits or honey.
10. Eat only permitted foods. The basis of a healthy diet should be vegetables, fruits, cereals. Keep a balance of proteins, fats, carbohydrates.
11. Serve with balsamic vinegar, lemon or lime juice to speed up and improve digestion.
12. Minimize salt intake, it helps retain excess fluid in the body.

**Allowed and forbidden foods**

The ration of the models consists of healthy foods with low calories. Breakfast and lunch should consist of foods rich with protein and complex carbohydrates. In the afternoon, choose vegetables, sweet and sour fruits and berries. Pineapples should be consumed as often as possible, these fruits contribute to fat burning due to the proteolytic enzyme - bromelain. Here is a table of acceptable product of models diet:

| Allowed foods | Calories (kcal) | Proteins, g | Carbohydrates, g | Fats, g |
|---|---|---|---|---|
| Vegetables and greens | | | | |
| Cauliflower | 29 | 2.6 | 5.6 | 0.4 |
| Broccoli cabbage | 30 | 2.9 | 4.1 | 0.5 |
| Cabbage Brussels sprouts | 42 | 4.8 | 7.9 | - |
| Artichoke | 27 | 1.2 | 5.9 | 0.1 |
| Iceberg lettuce | 15 | 0.9 | 1.9 | 0.1 |
| Sweet pepper | 30 | 1.3 | 5.2 | - |
| Parsley | 46 | 3.7 | 7.5 | 0.4 |
| Arugula | 24 | 2.6 | 2 | 0.7 |
| Asparagus | 19 | 1.9 | 2.9 | 0.1 |
| Carrots | 31 | 1.3 | 7 | 0.1 |
| Beets | 50 | 1.8 | 10.2 | - |
| Cucumber | 16 | 0.8 | 2.9 | - |
| Tomato | 19 | 0.6 | 4.3 | 0.2 |
| Fruit | | | | |
| Pineapple | 50 | 0.4 | 10.5 | 0.2 |
| Grapefruit | 30 | 0.7 | 6.4 | 0.2 |
| Lemon | 15 | 0.9 | 2.9 | 0.1 |
| Lime | 15 | 0.9 | 2.9 | 0.1 |
| Pomegranate | 51 | 0.9 | 13.8 | - |
| Baked apples | 90 | 0.5 | 24.2 | 0.3 |
| Cereals and cereals | | | | |
| Wild rice | 102 | 4 | 21.3 | 0.3 |
| Buckwheat porridge on water | 91 | 3.2 | 17, 2 | 0.8 |
| Oatmeal on water | 89 | 3 | 15.1 | 1.8 |
| Millet groats on water | 93 | 3 | 17.2 | 0.8 |
| Dressings and seasonings | | | | |
| Ginger | 81 | 1.8 | 15.7 | 0.9 |
| Balsamic vinegar | 87 | 0.5 | 17, 1 | - |
| Dairy products | | | | |
| Skim milk | 32 | 2 | 4.9 | 0.1 |
| buttermilk 0% fat | 31 | 3 | 3.7 | 0.1 |
| Skimmed cottage cheese | 72 | 16.5 | 1.2 | - |
| Meat and eggs | | | | |
| Chicken fillet | 138 | 32 | 0.4 | 1.7 |
| Eggs ku Soft boiled fish | 160 | 12.9 | 0.7 | 11.9 |
| Omelet | 185 | 9.8 | 2 | 15.7 |
| Vegetable fats | | | | |
| Olive oil | 897 | - | - | 100 |

A slender figure with perfect body contours is everyday work. To maintain beautiful forms, you will have to strictly monitor the diet, observe the diet rules of models, and completely eliminate high-calorie foods. Wishing to remain always slim should avoid the following foods:

| Prohibited foods | Calories (kcal) | Proteins, g | Carbohydrates, g | Fats, g |
|---|---|---|---|---|
| **Vegetables and greens** | | | | |
| Corn | 102 | 3.4 | 15.7 | 0.4 |
| Potatoes | 79 | 1.9 | 18.2 | 2.9 |
| **Fruits and berries** | | | | |
| Bananas | 94 | 1.4 | 21.9 | 0.2 |
| Grapes | 64 | 0.7 | 16.9 | 0.2 |
| **Flour and pasta** | | | | |
| Spaghetti | 345 | 10.3 | 71.4 | 1.1 |
| Pasta | 378 | 10.3 | 69.8 | 1, 1 |
| Pasta | 343 | 10.1 | 71.4 | 1.1 |
| Dumplings | 156 | 7.7 | 18.9 | 2.5 |
| **Bakery products** | | | | |
| Baton | 263 | 7.4 | 50.8 | 3 |
| Baguette | 261 | 7.4 | 51.3 | 3 |
| Buns | 316 | 7.1 | 51, 2 | 6.3 |
| Bread | 228 | 7.6 | 46.3 | 1.9 |
| Pita | 272 | 8.2 | 57.2 | 0.8 |
| **Confectionery** | | | | |
| Caramel | 360 | - | 98 | 0.1 |
| Chocolate candies | 451 | 4.4 | 67.4 | 19.9 |
| Corn sticks | 324 | 8.2 | 75.1 | 1.3 |
| Cookies | 416 | 7.4 | 75 | 11.9 |
| Gingerbread | 363 | 5.7 | 71.5 | 6.4 |
| Cakes | 396 | 3.7 | 47.2 | 22 5 |
| Shortbread dough | 402 | 6.4 | 50 | 21.5 |
| Sweet crackers | 396 | 10.2 | 73.7 | 2.1 |
| Jam | 237 | 0.2 | 56.6 | 0.1 |
| **Sauces and seasonings** | | | | |
| Lean Mayonnaise | 203 | 1.4 | 4.7 | 19.5 |
| Ketchup | 92 | 1.7 | 22.3 | 1 |
| Honey | 330 | 0.7 | 81.4 | - |
| Sugar | 397 | - | 100 | - |
| **Alcohol-containing drinks** | | | | |
| Sweet wine | 81 | - | 5.1 | - |
| Cognac | 240 | - | 0.1 | - |
| Vodka | 236 | - | 0.1 | - |
| Beer | 43 | 0.2 | 4.9 | - |

## Pros and cons

Each diet has its negative and positive points, the model diet is no exception . In addition, strict food restriction is not suitable for everyone. Low-calorie diets are contraindicated for lactating mothers and pregnant women, as well as people engaged in hard physical labor or suffering from diseases of the digestive system. Before embarking on a three or seven-day course of getting rid of extra pounds, consider the pros and cons of the diet of supermodels:

## Advantages

- guaranteed result in a short time;
- affordable products that do not require large cash costs or special culinary skills.

## Disadvantages

- unbalanced diet, the body does not receive all the necessary substances;
- attacks of hunger, which can lead to a breakdown.

## The menu of the models diet

Dishes are cooking with the maximum preservation of valuable substances. The vegetables are cooked steamed, so they are tastier and healthier. Porridge is boiled in water to make it low-calorie. Salads season with sour fruit juices to speed up metabolism. A highly effective model diet for 7 days implies the right combination of products. Protein food is better absorbed when consumed alone or with vegetables and herbs. Complex carbohydrates need to be combined with salads. Fat is completely discarded for the period of the diet or minimized consumption.

## For 3 days

A short-term model diet for 3 days is used in emergency cases when it is necessary to quickly reduce body volume. Used no more than once every 30 days. After 16 hours it is forbidden to eat, only water drinking. If you use the liquid in a heated form, then the feeling of hunger dulls. It is recommended to drink herbal decoctions, but without sweeteners. A three-day express course is strict and gentle. Extreme 3-day weight loss course:

- Breakfast (first) - 1 hard boiled egg.
- Breakfast (second) - 150 grams of low fat cottage cheese and green tea.
- Lunch - 150 g of cottage cheese with 0% fat and herbal tea.

The gentle option will also give positive results, maybe 1-2 kilograms less. Moderate three-day diet of top models:

- Breakfast - 2 soft-boiled eggs or 150 grams of porridge (buckwheat, oat, millet) on the water.
- Lunch - 100 grams of steamed fish and 300 g of salad from any green vegetables. It is allowed to replace fish with chicken fillet (100 g) or low-fat cottage cheese (150 g). A dietary salad can be prepared from several types of herbs and seasoned with lemon juice or balsamic vinegar.
- Afternoon snack - a cup of green tea, 2 non-nutritious fruits. Fresh fruits are allowed to be replaced with a handful of dried fruits.
- Dinner I - 2 slices of rye bread with butter or curd with zero percent fat, herbal tea.
- Dinner II - a decoction of soothing herbs.

## For 7 days

The Weekly Models Diet cannot be carried out more often than once every 60 days. You must eat a variety of foods, so the diet may be used as an emergency measure to reduce body volume. To sustain such a period not every girl can do. Salvation from hunger attacks during the 7-day diet is green tea, which gives vigor and dulls appetite. To strengthen the process of losing weight, it is replaced by a decoction of herbs that have a fat-burning effect. An approximate menu of models for every day during the week (option No. 1):

- breakfast: buckwheat porridge on water - 150 g; green vegetable salad with parsley seasoned with lemon juice;
- lunch: stewed cauliflower - 200 g; 1 soft-boiled egg; a slice of rye bread with curd;
- afternoon tea: green tea; medium-sized grapefruit;
- dinner: rice (100 g) with stewed broccoli (150 g).

You can combine the ingredients at your own discretion. A slight increase in serving size is not critical. The main thing is to use only permitted products with low calorie content (option No. 2):

- breakfast: barley porridge on the water - 150 g; white cabbage salad with cucumber and herbs, seasoned with balsamic vinegar;
- lunch: vegetable soup without potatoes - 250 ml; hard-boiled egg (2 pieces); a piece of rye bread;

- afternoon tea: herbal tea; pineapple - 150 g;
- dinner: buckwheat (100 g) with stewed cauliflower (150 g).

## Exit from the models diet

A sharp change in diet is stress for the body. During a low-calorie diet, not only the breakdown of fats occurs, but also the cleansing of toxins of the whole body. If You after the end of the diet, abruptly begin to eat the usual refined food from supermarkets, have a bite of dry food, and drink alcohol, then you can significantly disrupt the digestion process.

**Recommendations for the correct exit from the diet of supermodels:**

- return to an ordinary diet gradually;
- review the diet, eliminate harmful foods forever, and not just for the period of the diet;
- start the fourth or eighth day after limiting the diet with light meals (salads, cereals on the water, fruits, vegetables, etc.);
- continue to observe the drinking regimen in order to maintain a normal metabolism and release the body from harmful substances;
- eat fractionally, in small portions.

# Low-carb diets
## Diet by glycemic index

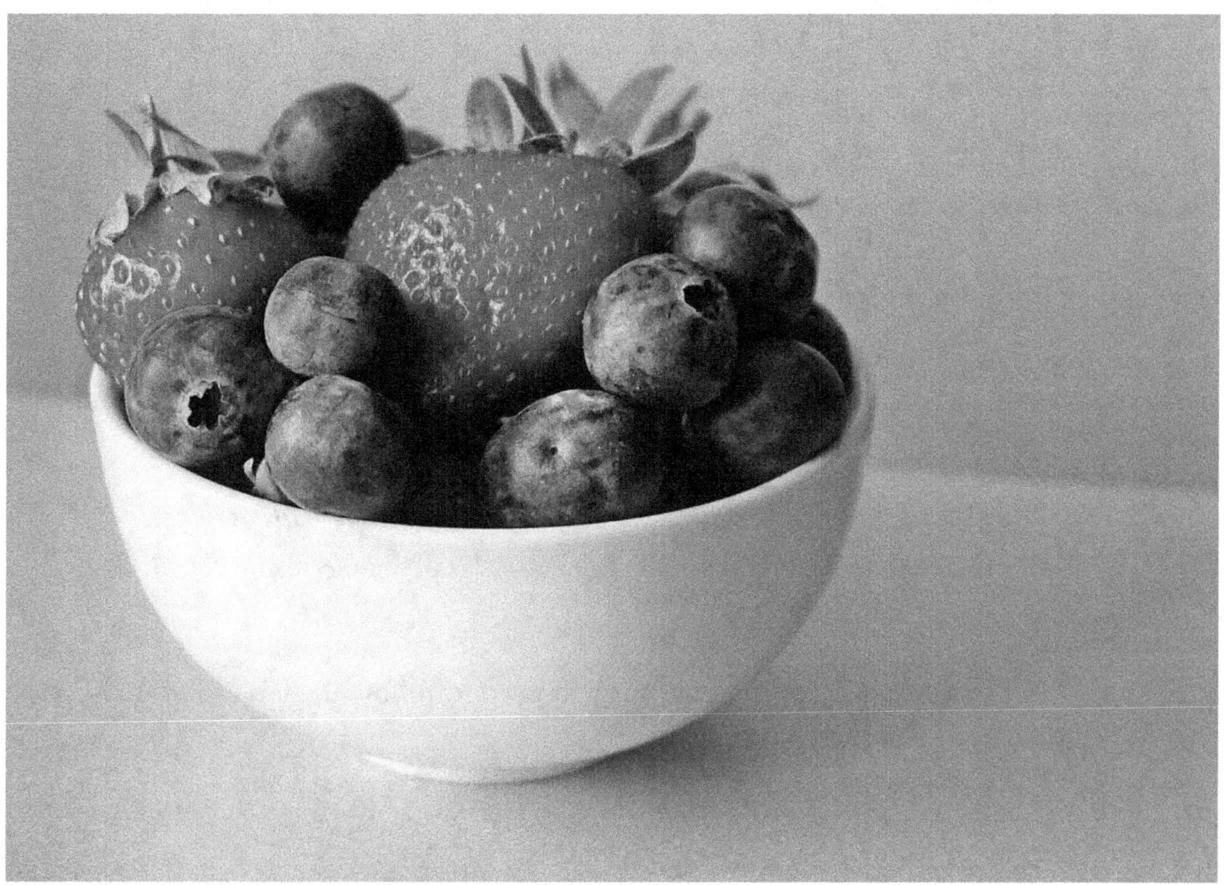

**Diet by glycemic index: menu and table of products**

Features of the course of chemical reactions can not only build the body, but also prevent obesity, metabolic syndrome, diabetes mellitus, gastrointestinal and cardiovascular diseases. For that is designed a low-carb diet, which is based on nutrition at the glycemic index (GI) of foods.

**What is the glycemic index?**

The term reflects the rate of conversion of carbohydrates into glucose. Blood sugar and insulin production depend on this. Then lower is the GI of the product, then slower glucose is absorbed.

It leads to a violation of metabolic processes in the tissues. As a result, a person receives too much energy, which does not have time to be spent and is saved "in reserve" in problem areas of the body.

## The essence of a hypoglycemic diet

This nutrition system involves the use of complex carbohydrates - foods with low GI. The body receives the necessary energy, fat breakdown occurs, excess weight disappears.



It does not have strict dietary restrictions, but you need to follow the tables' information that indicate of GI of a particular product.

## Efficiency

In 2 weeks, the glycemic diet helps to lose up to 5 kg of excess weight. Weight loss is due to the burning of fat cells.

## Indications and contraindications

This system is suitable for:

- those who constantly experience a feeling of hunger and can not adhere to strict diets;
- wishing to reduce the amount of "bad" cholesterol, strengthen the immune system
- people who switch to proper nutrition.

The glycemic diet affects the entire circulatory system, so it has serious limitations:

- mental disorders;
- varicose veins and other diseases of the circulatory system;
- ulcer, gastritis;
- pathology of the heart;
- period of pregnancy and lactation.

*Children and the elderly are not allowed to follow the diet*

So that insulin deficiency does not provoke severe consequences, they need to gradually reduce the glycemic load. Doctors do not advise diabetics to follow this diet due to the fact that few studies are conducted in the field of dietary restriction.

## Nutrition Rules

Glycemic index diet has options.

1. The basis of the diet is products with a low glycemic index.
2. Simple carbohydrates, sweets, and alcohol are excluded from the diet at the time of weight loss.
3. The daily calorie content of dishes for healthy weight loss is at least 1500 kcal.
4. The food is steamed, consumed in baked, boiled, stewed, but not fried form.
5. Fractional nutrition includes 5 meals a day (3 main and 2 snacks).
6. The optimal serving size is 200 g. Overeating or a strong feeling of hunger should not be allowed.
7. Drinking regimen should be at least 30 ml of pure water per 1 kg of weight.
8. In addition to the diet, cardio loads are recommended - running, swimming, aerobics. They speed up the burning of fat.

## Glycemic index

| Snacks | Index | Starch products | Index |
|---|---|---|---|
| Pizza | 33 | White flour | 33 |
| Chocolate | 49 | White rice | 38 |
| Cupcake | 54 | Spaghetti | 38 |
| Popcorn | 55 | Potato | 44 |
| Energy bar | 58 | White bread | 49 |
| Lemonade | 72 | Brown rice | 55 |
| Donut | 76 | Pancakes | 67 |
| Jelly candies | 80 | Rye bread | 80 |
| Crackers | 83 | Baked Potatoes | 85 |

| Vegetables | Index | Fruits | Index |
|---|---|---|---|
| Broccoli | 10 | Cherries | 22 |
| Pepper | 10 | Apples | 38 |
| Salad | 10 | Oranges | 43 |
| Mushrooms | 10 | Grapes | 46 |
| Cucumbers | 10 | Kiwi | 52 |
| Green Peas | 48 | Bananas | 56 |
| Carrots | 49 | Pineapples | 66 |
| Beets | 64 | Melon | 72 |
| Onions | 75 | Dates | 103 |

| Dairy Products | Index |
|---|---|
| Yogurt without additives | 14 |
| Skim yogurt | 14 |
| Milk | 30 |
| Soy milk | 31 |
| Ryazhenka | 49 |
| Kako | 32 |
| Yogurt with | 36 |
| Custard | 43 |
| Ice cream | 60 |

The nutrition system is based on dividing all carbohydrate-products into groups. A glycemic score of up to 39 units is considered low. This food contains the so-called "slow" carbohydrates. **These products include:**

| Product name | Glycemic index |
|---|---|
| Brussels sprouts, cauliflower, broccoli | 15 |
| Cucumbers, bell peppers | 15 |
| Natural yogurt without additives | 20 |
| Dark chocolate (at least 85% cocoa) | 20 |
| Berries (raspberries, cherries, blackberries, strawberries, blueberries ) | 25 |
| Tomatoes, carrots | 30 |
| Milk | 30 |
| Whole grain bread | 35 |
| Apples | 35 |

40–69 is considered to be average.

**Examples of products:**

| Product name | Glycemic index |
|---|---|
| Oat flakes | 40 |
| Coconuts | 45 |
| Pasta of durum wheat | 50 |
| Pineapple | 50 |
| Peaches | 50 |
| Ketchup, mustard | 55 |
| Dlinnozernovoy Figure | 60 |
| Pizza cheese | 60 |
| Boiled potatoes | 65 |
| Rye bread | 65 |

## High glycemic index of foods with a mark "70" and above:

| Product name | Glycemic index |
|---|---|
| Milk chocolate | 70 |
| Pearl barley, semolina | 70 |
| Zucchini | 75 |
| Waffles | 75 |
| Mashed potatoes | 80 |
| Unsweetened pastries | 85 |
| Wheat bread | 90 |
| Baked or fried potatoes | 95 |
| Toast bread | 100 |
| Beer | 110 |

## Low-glycemic diet menu :

- breakfast - oatmeal on water with scrambled eggs or cottage cheese, salad with butter, unsweetened tea;
- snack - fruit, nuts or cheese;
- lunch - brown rice, beef stroganoff with mushrooms, cucumber and tomato salad with olive oil dressing;
- afternoon tea - natural yogurt;
- dinner - shrimp salad.

When creating a menu with a low glycemic index, consider these recommendations:

- Include in your diet your favorite foods from the low GI list. This will help maintain a positive mood during the diet.
- Once a day, eat a dish with average glycemic indicators.

**Advantages and disadvantages of the GI nutritional system**

Advantages of the glycemic index diet:

- A balanced diet does not lead to starvation.
- The lost pounds do not come back, because fat is gone, and not excess water and muscle.
- Healthy eating habits are formed, a gradual transition to proper nutrition occurs.

Among the disadvantages are the following:

- It is necessary to remember the glycemic indicators of the products.
- The result appears gradually - after 1-3 months of diet.
- Such nutrition affects the circulatory system of the body. Before starting a diet, consult a doctor.
- Keep a balance - if you ate a high-calorie dish, add foods with a low index to other meals.
- Do not exclude proteins from the diet, with minimal GI they are important for building muscle. Proteins are found in lean meats, fish, dairy and fermented milk products without sugar.
- "Correct" fats, which stabilize the functioning of the female genital organs, should be up to 30% of the total diet. These nutrients are found in nuts, eggs, avocados, olive oil and whole milk.

# Ketogenic diet

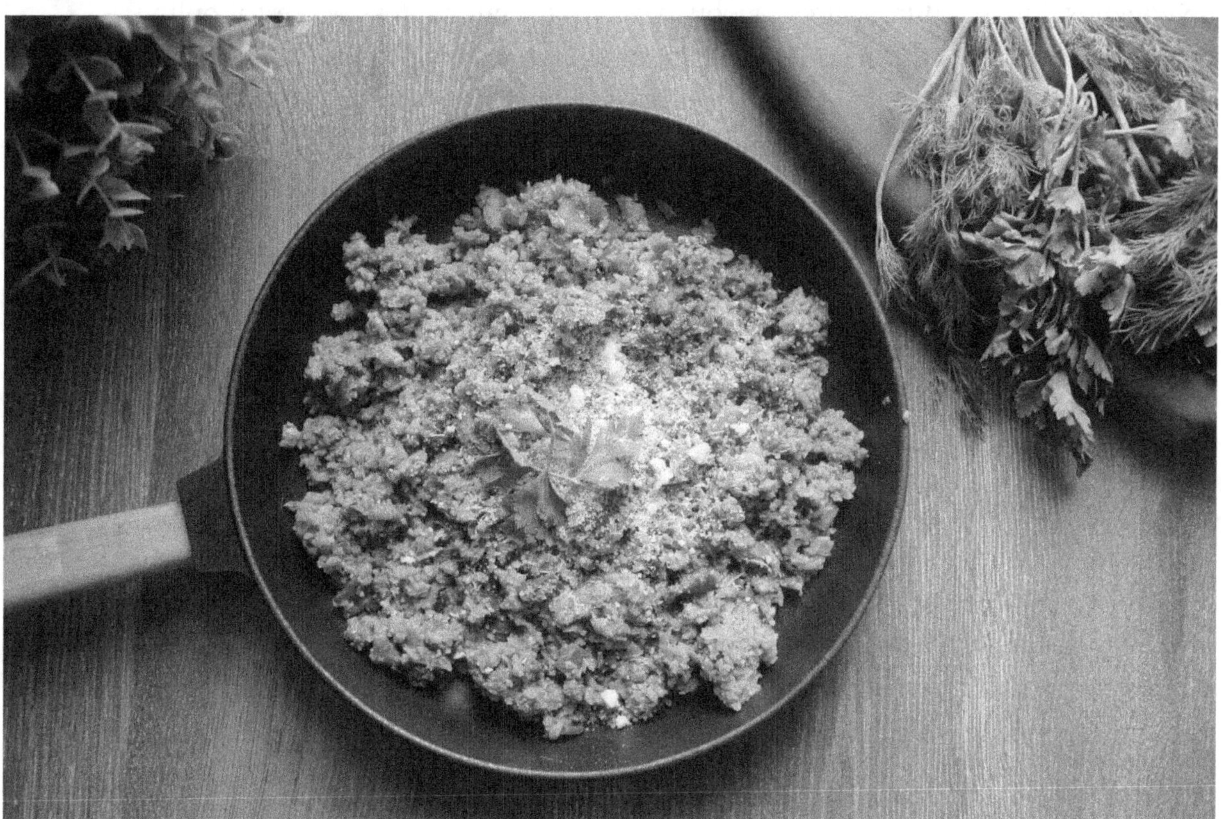

**Ketogenic diet: a menu for weight loss.**

A diet based on avoiding carbohydrates and increasing fat intake still causes a lot of controversy among its adherents and nutritionists. A ketogenic diet promises that with strict adherence to the rules, with moderate physical activity per month, you can lose up to 10 kilograms of fat and gain lean muscle mass. Largely thanks to this statement, the diet has become popular among athletes, bodybuilders and those who want to lose weight quickly.

**What is a ketogenic diet?**

The ketogenic principle of nutrition by construction is largely similar to the popular low-carb diet or paleo-diet. Initially, this eating pattern was used to treat children who have epilepsy. Today, the technique has gained wide popularity and is actively used by women for weight loss, athletes to dry the body and build muscle.

The essence of ketogenic nutrition is to minimize carbohydrate intake, replacing lack of high fat and moderate protein. The carbohydrates that are ingested are processed by the body into glucose, most of which is used to feed the brain, and insulin is a substance necessary for the conversion of glucose into useful energy (a universal energy source that takes part in all biochemical processes).

Glucose accumulates in subcutaneous fat and muscle in the form of glucose-6-phosphate dehydrogenase or glycogen. Since in its pure form it is used as primary energy, deferred glycogen is converted into subcutaneous fat and it accumulates. When following a ketogenic diet, the body smoothly transitions to a state better known as ketosis. It occurs in pregnant and newborn children. Artificially, a condition can be caused by turning to high-fat or carbohydrate-free nutrition.

**The process of ketosis**

When the body begins to experience a shortage of carbohydrates, the liver converts fat cells into acetyl coenzyme A, a compound used in the biochemical reactions of the Krebs cycle. This substance reacts with oxaloacetate, during which it is broken down into ketone bodies - beta-hydroxybutyrate, acetoacetic acid and acetone. This natural process helps the body survive hunger.

With a prolonged glucose deficiency, the body gradually turns into a state where intensive production of ketone bodies begins to occur automatically, then you can officially declare that the person is in a state of ketosis. Ketone bodies penetrate the blood-brain barrier, nourish brain cells in conditions of "starvation", improve mental performance, increase endurance.

**The Difference between a Ketogenic and a Low-Carb Diet**

A superficial examination of a ketogenic diet may seem very similar to a carbohydrate-free diet, but in fact they have some differences. A low-carb diet suggests that you refuse to eat "heavy" carbohydrates, replacing them with fiber. With a ketogenic diet, the total amount of carbohydrates decreases, against the background of increased consumption of vegetable or animal fats and foods with a moderate protein content.

During a low-carb diet, the body enters a state of ketosis only for a while, and when you exit, you may feel severe emotional discomfort, depressed, overwhelmed. Ketogenic nutrition suggests that ketone bodies will remain in the body continuously, which significantly reduces the risk of severe stress for the body.

Another difference can be seen if you conduct a simple diagnostic test. Buy special test strips from the pharmacy to determine your blood ketone level. With a ketogenic diet, the level of beta-hydroxybutyrate will be between 0.5–3 mM / L. Low-carb diets only partially limit the amount of carbohydrates, so the level of beta-hydroxybutyrate will never reach such levels.

**Advantages of ketogenic diet**

Most people can not only safely use the keto method from time to time, but also observe its principles on a regular basis. The main advantages include:

- Effective weight loss and improved muscle relief. The advantages for losing weight on a keto diet are obvious - the body uses subcutaneous fat as an alternative energy source. At the same time, the effect of this method of losing weight remains even a long time after leaving the diet.
- Lowering blood sugar and lowering insulin resistance. Ketogenic nutrition helps to lower blood sugar, therefore it is often prescribed by doctors for the treatment and prevention of diabetes. In addition, many studies show that low-carb foods help people lower their blood insulin levels to normal levels.
- Improving mental performance and a surge of strength. At first, switching to nutrition without carbohydrates, you will feel weakness, drowsiness. So the body adapts to new circumstances. After a time when the level of ketone bodies in the blood rises, you will notice that your working capacity has increased.
- Normalization of nutrition behavior. The ketogenic method helps fight metabolic syndrome, a disease that increases the risk of developing obesity, heart failure, and type 2 diabetes.
- Lowering cholesterol and normalizing blood pressure. A ketogenic diet normalizes the level of triglycerides and other components of the lipid profile, can positively affect the level of lipoproteins, which will benefit patients with cardiovascular diseases.

**What diseases are effective ?**

A ketogenic diet is used for weight loss and muscle drying in sports, but it also has many other advantages. According to European scientists, this principle of nutrition helps in the treatment and prevention of diseases:

- nervous system. A low-carb diet significantly improves the psycho-emotional state of patients with severe neurological pathologies. Helps reduce symptoms of Alzheimer's, Parkinson's disease, epilepsy.
- Oncological problems. A ketogenic diet increases the effectiveness of anti-cancer therapy, so it is often prescribed to patients who have malignant tumors.
- Acne and dermatitis. The exclusion of all harmful products from the diet helps to

cure inflammation of the skin, remove redness, and reduce the number of rashes.

- Polycystic ovary. This disease has a direct relationship with insulin levels, so switching to low-carb ketogenic nutrition increases the chances of successful treatment.

## Types of diet

Each person is individual and this applies not only to moral principles, character, but also to other indicators: physique, nutritional preferences, body characteristics. The developers of the ketogenic system took this fact into account and developed several nutritional schemes that help people with different body masses achieve high weight loss results. In total, there are 4 schemes for low-carb behavior:

- Standard diet (SKD) involves eating a large amount of fat, moderate protein and minimizing carbohydrates.
- Cyclic ketogenic diet (CKD). Its meaning is to eat low-carb foods for the first 5 days, and only high-carb meals for the next two days.
- Directional or Targeted Nutrition Scheme (NKD) has been developed specifically for athletes. It should follow standard rules, but consume carbohydrates in food to increase stamina before and after training.
- The high-protein approach is very similar to the standard low-carb diet with some differences. The level of carbohydrates and fats remains the same, but the amount of protein rises to 35%.

## Reasons for effectiveness

There is much debate about the appropriateness of following a ketogenic diet, but scientific evidence inexorably proves its effectiveness compared to traditional low-fat nutritional schemes. It was found that people who lose weight using this technique lose 2 times more kilograms of excess weight than those who are counting calories or follow nutrition by points. There are several reasons for this phenomenon:

- The body will not receive the usual source of fuel - carbohydrates, therefore it will not save energy "in reserve".
- The fats and proteins that enter the body are processed into ketone bodies. With constant ketosis, a person has an increased desire to work, play sports, which means it burns more calories.
- Ketogenic nutritional technique helps to normalize metabolism, affects the level of leptin and ghrelin - hormones that are responsible for human nutritional behavior.

## Ketogenic diet for weight loss

According to the standard diet, 70-75% of the daily calories must be obtained from fats, 5% from carbohydrates and 10-15 from proteins. These norms must be observed in order to enter and stay at the level of ketosis for the required period. At the same time, experts emphasize that some people can expand the carbohydrate ratio to 12% and still remain in a ketotic state.

For weight loss, the emphasis should be on fats. It is strictly forbidden to abuse proteins. In large doses, they can break down to glucose (the so-called gluconeogenesis process), slowing down the process of ketosis. Calculate the protein norm in accordance with your weight: for every kilogram of body weight per day, there should be no more than 1.8 grams of protein.

It is worth considering that the rules that may differ slightly for each person, therefore, for an accurate calculation of individual needs, you should contact sports nutrition specialists or doctors. They will calculate the norm, based on your d calorie consumption, age, hormonal background, lifestyle, and physique.

## The list of allowed products

It depends on what you will eat: how quickly you will enter the state of ketosis and how long you can hold on to it. A ketogenic diet contains lists of allowed and prohibited foods. You can eat:

- All types of meat (poultry, pork, beef, lamb), ham, sausages, eggs. It will be better if these products are home-made.
- Fish and seafood. The ideal choice would be fatty fish varieties such as salmon, trout, herring. Consuming shrimp, squid, mussels is welcome. It is advisable to cook these products without bread crumbs.
- Vegetables. Preference should be given to green vegetables. It is allowed to eat tomatoes, sweet peppers, onions, eggplant, spinach, cucumbers, pumpkins. Root crops such as beets, parsnips or carrots are available in limited quantities.
- Fatty dairy and sour-milk products - cream, cottage cheese, butter, milk, goat cheese. Be wary of fermented milk products with flavorings, it is better to buy natural homemade or whole milk.
- Nuts, seeds, mushrooms.
- Fermented products - yogurt, sourdough, sauerkraut, buttermilk.
- Dietary oils - olive, linseed, coconut, almond. You should choose unrefined first-pressed oils.

- Natural fats - lard, ghee.
- Spices - basil, dill, parsley and more.

## What foods are prohibited

The more restrictions on carbohydrates you allow yourself, the faster the process of losing weight will begin. All high-carb products are strictly prohibited. Small exceptions are berries, avocados, guacamole and carambola, dark chocolate with cocoa more than 70% - they can be eaten in moderation. Other prohibited foods include:

- Sugar and starch. You need to refuse white or milk chocolate, any baking, rolls, ice cream, desserts, cookies or pastries, breakfast cereals and granola.
- Margarine, refined oils. They contain a large number of omega-6 acids and trans fats, doubtful on use. Under the ban - soybean, corn, sunflower, rapeseed oil, mayonnaise.
- Fruits or dried fruits. They contain a lot of fructose, sucrose and other sugar derivatives. The only exceptions are sour berries, strawberries, coconut and avocados.
- Legumes - peas, beans, lentils. The only exceptions are chickpeas and green bean pods.
- Cereals - rye, barley, wheat (pasta, noodles) and other cereals.

## Drinks and alcohol

It is strictly forbidden to drink fruit juices (even if they are natural), sweet soda and mineral water with gas. Alcohol is not recommended. The only exceptions are dry red wines, unsweetened cocktails and spirits (gin, rum, vodka, whiskey) in moderation. The basis of the drinking diet should be:

- clean water;
- all types of tea;
- herbal decoctions to your taste;
- cocoa, stevia;
- natural coffee (it is appreciated if you will drink it with the addition of cream).

## Menus for the week

Start a ketogenic diet with a clearly designed action plan and menu. When drawing up the diet, keep in mind that you will have to starve for the first day. Allowed to drink only water. This is necessary in order for the body to completely use up all glucose stores and begin to develop ketone bodies. After a week, it is advisable to interrupt the process of losing weight so that the body recovers itself and normalizes carbohydrate metabolism.

For weight loss, you need to repeat the cycle 2-3 times. During this time, you can lose from 5 to 15 kilograms. For an example, take such a menu for a week:

| | **Breakfast** | **Lunch** | **Afternoon Snack** | **Dinner** |
|---|---|---|---|---|
| **Day 1** | Omelet of three eggs with bacon and tomatoes. Tea with milk without sugar. | Portion of brussels sprouts soup with mushrooms. Boiled chicken breast with stewed eggplant and bell pepper - 200 g. | Almonds 40 g, 2 slices of cheese. | Fresh vegetable salad with sour cream (200 g). 200 gram salmon steak with spices and lemon. A glass of buttermilk. |
| **Day 2** | Fat homemade yogurt or sourdough with nuts. A cup of natural coffee with cream. | Beef broth with egg - 1 serving. Braised beef in tomato sauce - 150 g. Sauerkraut salad with olive oil and onions - 150 g. A | Fat yogurt. | Fish stewed in sour cream with onions. 200 grams of brown rice. Tea. |
| **Day 3** | Fried eggs from three eggs with bell pepper. Coffee with cream. | Ear (without potatoes and other prohibited ingredients) - 1 serving. Beefsteak with stewed cabbage - 200 g. | Cottage cheese with sour cream - 100 g. | Chicken breast, baked in the oven with cream and broccoli - 250 g. |
| **Day 4** | One apple, 50 g walnuts, black tea with milk, yogurt - 100 g. | Filet turkey with cranberry sauce - 150 g. A portion of stewed zucchini. | Fat yogurt. | Greek salad - 150 g. Fried fish - 150 g. A Cup of milk. |
| **Day 5** | Protein shake - 1 cup, a handful of nuts. | Soup with chickpeas - 200 ml. Coffee with cream, cheese - 50 g. | Fermented baked milk- 1 cup. | Beef stew with vegetables - 200 g. 2 cottage cheese pancakes with sour cream and a rosehip broth. |
| **Day 6** | 100 g of cottage cheese casserole. An Apple. Mug of coffee with cream. | Rabbit stewed with sour cream - 150 g. Asparagus - 100 g. Borsch - 100 g (without potatoes). | Fermented baked milk- 1 cup. , 30 g almonds. | Vegetable stew - 1 serving. Chicken leg - 80-100 g. Tea. |
| **Day 7** | Two-egg omelet with spinach. Coffee with cream. | Meat broth with meatballs (without flour and potatoes) - 1 serving. Beef Azu with cabbage - 150 g. | Yogurt with nuts - 80 g. | Seafood and parmesan salad - 150 g. Cottage cheese casserole - 100 g. Rosehip broth. |

## How to achieve a state of ketosis

American developers of a ketogenic diet argue that achieving a state of ketosis is simple. To do this, observe a amount of points:

1. Limit carbohydrate intake. Do not think that you need to remove complex carbohydrates from the diet. If you want to achieve really good results, you should reduce the intake of all types of carbohydrates to 35 grams per day.

2. Monitor protein intake. Too much protein can cause the production of additional glucose, which is highly undesirable for the ketogenic principle of nutrition.

3. Fats obtained with food are not converted to extra pounds. If you think differently, then you are deeply mistaken. Due to a lack of carbohydrates, the body converts fats into energy.

4. Drink plenty of fluids. This will help control electrolyte balance. It is advisable to drink up to four liters of fluid per day.

5. Stop making unplanned snacks. The diet should go on schedule. If you want to lose weight, categorically refuse street food.

6. Start following the ketogenic weight loss technique with fasting.

7. For maximum effect, add exercise to your diet. Consider options for light fitness, outdoor walks, group exercises in the pool. Practice the sport for 20-30 minutes a day.

## Adaptation period

You can find out that everything was done correctly by analyzing with special test strips. Another way is to carefully look at changes in health status. In the early days, the following symptoms of ketosis may appear:

1. Frequent urination. Keto nutrition acts like good diuretic medications. With urine, the body tries to get rid of ketone bodies and acetoacetate.

2. Dry mouth. Frequent urination leads to dehydration, so thirst is a normal process. Try to drink plenty of fluids while replenishing your salt, potassium, magnesium, sodium, and other electrolytes.

3. Bad breath. One of the ketone bodies - acetone - is partially secreted through the respiratory tract. When breathing, others may smell overripe fruits or nail polish removers. Unpleasant aroma is a temporary phenomenon.

The appearance of such symptoms indicates that the process of losing weight has begun, and you are overcoming a period called keto-flu. After the adaptation process is completed, the negative reactions of the body disappear, you will experience a surge of vigor and strength, and your appetite will decrease. To reduce unpleasant phenomena, you can start taking vitamins, be sure to drink more liquid. On average, adaptation takes from 4 to 5 days.

**Possible consequences and side effects**

Ketogenic diet suggests that you follow all the recommendations - reduce carbohydrate intake, increase the amount of fat. Be sure to drink about four liters of fluid per day. Adverse reactions often occur among beginners and are more associated with dehydration or lack of vitamins. Make sure you drink and eat good micronutrient foods. Of the adverse reactions, the appearance of:

- Convulsions is a sign of magnesium deficiency. Often cramps prevail at night or in the morning. To get rid of them, experts recommend replenishing the water-salt balance and taking supplements with omega-3 acids.
- Constipation. A common cause of its occurrence is dehydration. The solution is to increase fluid intake. If this does not help, you should use probiotics or increase fiber intake.
- Fast heartbeat. Start taking multivitamins with potassium and magnesium, dietary supplements with creatine monohydrate.
- The appearance of dyspepsia is an upset stomach, acid belching, heartburn. If such symptoms appear, it is worth trying a little to limit fat intake.
- Itching, scabies. They appear due to skin irritation with acetone, which leaves the body with sweat. Try to take a shower more often, choose clothes that do not fit the body.

**What is the danger of ketoacidosis**

There is an opinion that ketosis necessarily leads to the development of ketoacidosis - a condition associated with a violation of carbohydrate metabolism due to a lack of insulin. With ketoacidosis, blood acidity rises, and the body goes into a condition called metabolic acidosis. Due to acidic blood, internal organs cannot function normally, which can lead to serious consequences, up to a coma. The first signs of disorders are:

- severe vomiting;
- abdominal pains;
- dehydration;
- drowsiness;
- prostration;
- low blood pressure up to 90/60 mm RT. st .;
- increase in heart rate (over 100 heartbeats per minute).

Ketoacidosis is a serious disease and requires immediate treatment, but it can not be a consequence of the keto diet. More often, a similar condition develops in patients with congenital type 1 diabetes, and if patients have reduced sensitivity to insulin during type 2 diabetes. In non-diabetics, the disease occurs extremely rarely due to a sedentary lifestyle, addiction to unhealthy foods, and severe stress.

**Contraindications**

Ketogenic nutrition helps to quickly lose up to 15 kilograms of excess weight, but not everyone can follow this weight loss technique. Doctors categorically forbid to follow her rules:

- during pregnancy;
- nursing mothers;
- patients with diabetes;
- people with diseases of the liver, kidneys, gastrointestinal tract, cardiovascular system;
- children
- seniors

# LCHF diet

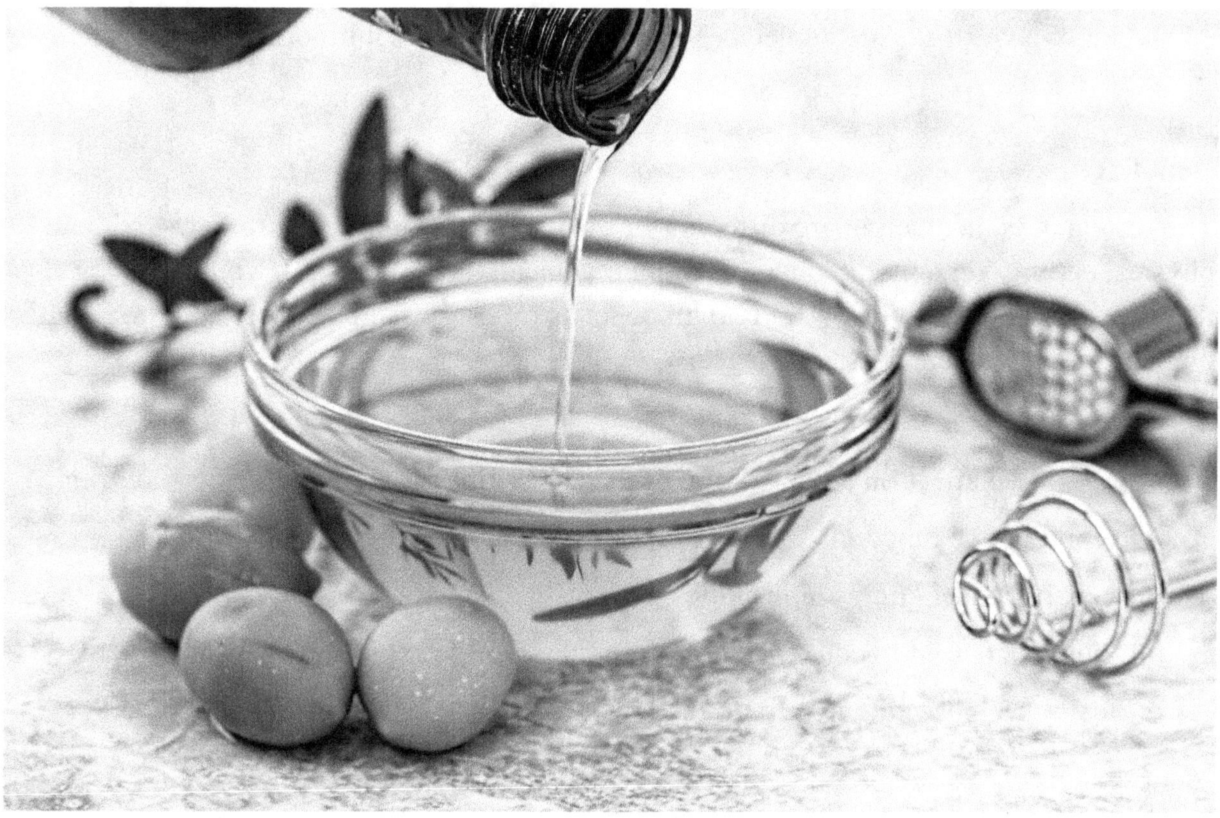

**LCHF diet for a week**

The abbreviation LCHF stands for Low Carb High Fat. High-fat diet promises not just fast, but rapid weight loss. Judging by the reviews, this technique does not cause drowsiness, apathy, irritability and hunger.

**How it works**

The LCHF diet is a low-carb diet, but it has several differences. Please note that there are 2 options for generating energy:

- Gluconeogenesis. This is getting energy through the utilization of proteins.
- Ketogenesis This is the name of the process of obtaining energy from adipose tissue, which decomposes during metabolism into ketone bodies.

Most low-carb diets focus on proteins. As a result, the body begins to receive energy due to gluconeogenesis. Excess protein food leads to kidney problems, deterioration of the skin, hair loss. The LCHF diet does not cause such side effects, since it focuses on fats. The mechanism of action of this technique is as follows:

1. When refusing carbohydrates, the body begins to rebuild.

2. As a result, fat breakdown products begin to be used for energy.

3. First, own stocks are depleted. Further, fats obtained with food are used.

## Benefits

The results of losing weight are different for everyone. Judging by the reviews, without physical activity for a month on a LCHF diet, you can throw 3-4 kg. If you play sports, then the plumb line will be 5-10 kg. It all depends on the initial body weight. The LCHF diet has several undeniable advantages:

- lack of hunger;
- a positive effect on the condition of the hair, skin, general well-being and even reproductive function;
- lack of sudden jumps in insulin;
- there is no need to consume large amounts of protein;
- losing weight without harm to the body.

## Basic rules

The LCHF diet, depending on the daily amount of carbohydrates, has three main options: strict (20–25 g), moderate (25–50 g), and liberal (50–100 g). The latter is suitable for those who train for several hours a week, are not overweight, do not get tired at the workplace and do not experience excruciating attacks of hunger. The high-fat, low-carb LCHF diet has a few more rules:

- menu taking into account the following proportions: fats - 70%, proteins - 20%, carbohydrates - 10%.
- Cook foods with minimal heat. Boiled, baked or steamed dishes are more useful than fried.
- Drink a glass of water half an hour before meals.

## List of foods for the LCHF diet

In a limited amount, the LCHF diet allows dark chocolate with 70% cocoa, coffee, tea, fruits, low-carb pasta. It is also allowed to introduce pumpkin, pickled vegetables, pastries from almond or coconut flour into the diet. The following products are allowed without exception:

| Product group Product | names |
|---|---|
| Meat | Bacon;<br>smoked meats;<br>beef;<br>sausages;<br>ham. |
| Sea fish | herring;<br>tuna;<br>salmon. |
| Oil | Olive;<br>sunflower;<br>flaxseed. |
| First courses of | fatty meat and fish broths. |
| Bird | duck;<br>goose;<br>a hen. |
| Vegetables "above ground" ,without starch | tomato;<br>green onions;<br>eggplant;<br>cucumber;<br>green beans;<br>zucchini;<br>zucchini;<br>cabbage. |
| Nuts | Flaxseed;<br>olives;<br>sesame;<br>walnuts;<br>cashew;<br>peanut. |

## Prohibited Foods

All simple carbohydrates must be banned. Only complex ones can be present in the diet, and in the amount indicated above. The following products are completely prohibited:

- sweet fermented milk products;

- carbonated drinks, kvass, beer;

- white bread, crackers from it;

- bakery products;

- cookies, cakes, waffles;

- pasta and bran;

- sugar;

- jam;

- chocolate, ice cream;

- root vegetables, including beets, potatoes, celery, carrots;

- fortified wines.

## LCHF Diet Menu for the Week

When choosing ingredients, do not trust the labels on the packages. The label "low-carb" or "complex carbohydrates" may be silent about the mix of starch, sweeteners, flour and sugar. This is important when formulating a diet . The sample menu might look like this:

| Day | Breakfast | Lunch | Dinner |
| --- | --- | --- | --- |
| 1 | omelet of 3-4 eggs; cucumber, tomato and mozzarella salad; cottage cheese with sour cream; coffee with cream. | coffee with cream; several pieces of cheese of different varieties. | grilled cheese; lamb shashlik; a glass of dry wine. |
| 2 | scrambled eggs with tomatoes and bacon; coffee with cream; cottage cheese with sour cream; salad of herbs, suluguni cheese and celery. | hard cheese; zucchini puree soup. | cheesecake with sun-dried tomatoes; tea with milk; a low-carb bread sandwich with soft cheese. |
| 3 | coffees with cream; cheesecakes with psyllium; sour cream 30%. | cauliflower fried in butter; chicken fillet with Bernese fatty sauce; salad of seasonal vegetables. | tea with milk; stewed chicken liver with creamy sauce; salad of nuts, tomato and onion with sour cream. |
| 4 | omelet with cheese and bacon; salad of mozzarella, arugula, spinach; coffee with cream. | zucchini pancakes with sour cream; pork with creamy sauce. | sweet pepper and tomato salad; suluguni cheese, smoked cheese, bacon. |
| 5 | cheese slices; scrambled eggs; steamed broccoli. | pumpkin puree; a sandwich made from low-carb bread and soft cheese. | a glass of red wine; grilled meat sausage; cutting vegetables. |
| 6 | cheese slices; fried eggs; coffee with milk. | steamed broccoli; beef steak; Sparkling water. | grilled meat with tomatoes and herbs; green tea. |
| 7 | scrambled eggs with tomatoes and sausage; cheese, salami; a handful of berries; coffee. | cheese slicing; seafood salad; Sparkling water. | steamed vegetables; Salmon steak; a glass of dry wine. |

**Side Effects**

During the first week, when switching to the LCHF diet, nausea, dizziness, and headache may occur. It gradually disappears when the body gets used to the new diet. If the diet was not formulated correctly, then the following side effects appear:

- osteoporosis;
- remineralization of bones;
- stones in the kidneys;
- avitaminosis;
- bloating;
- ketoacidosis;
- menstrual irregularities in women;
- increased cholesterol levels;
- dehydration;
- constipation, gastrointestinal disorders;
- pancreatitis.

**Contraindications**

*The LCHF diet is not recommended for the elderly as they are more likely to increase their cholesterol concentration.*

This can lead to atherosclerosis, and in the future - to stroke. Other contraindications to such a diet:

- diabetes mellitus;
- diseases of the heart and blood vessels;
- high cholesterol levels;
- lactation;
- pregnancy;
- frequent stresses;
- digestive disorders;
- menses.

**Recipes**

One of the benefits of the LCHF diet is the varied list of foods. Many recipes can be adapted to it. Nutritionists recommend increasing the number of apples and cabbage, as fiber helps to reduce the number of side effects when switching to a new diet.

**Cauliflower puree**
- Time: 40 minutes.
- Servings Per Container: 4 Persons.
- Difficulty: easy.

Instead of the usual potatoes, mashed cabbage is suitable as a side dish for meat dishes. The calorie content of the dish is about 33 kcal per 100 g. For the recipe, it is better to take not very large inflorescences.

Ingredients:

- butter - 3 tbsp.;
- head of cauliflower - 1 pc.;
- black pepper and salt - to taste;
- heavy cream - 1 cup;
- pine nuts - 1 handful.

Method of preparation:

1. Disassemble the cabbage into inflorescences, boil.
2. Drain the water, grind the vegetable into puree.
3. Add butter, cream, pepper, salt.
4. Sprinkle with toasted pine nuts on top.

**Coconut cookies**
- Time: 30 minutes.
- Servings Per Container: 2 Persons.
- Difficulty: easy.

Coconuts contain saturated fats that normalize cholesterol levels, thereby preventing atherosclerosis. Before making these cookies, you need to make sure that you are not allergic to coconut flour.

Ingredients:

- chicken egg - 1 pc .;
- coconut oil - 2 tbsp.;
- coconut flour - 2 tbsp.

Cooking method:

1. Mix all the ingredients, let the dough stand for a couple of minutes.
2. Form small cakes, spread on a baking sheet.
3. Bake for 10-12 minutes. at 180 degrees.

## LCHF Zucchini Pancakes

- Time: 50 minutes.
- Servings Per Container: 5 Persons.
- Difficulty: Medium.

To get sweet pancakes, you should add raisins, candied fruits, dried apricots or cottage cheese to them. Minced meat or fried mushrooms will help diversify the taste. These pancakes should be served with sour cream or garlic-cream sauce.

Ingredients:

- coconut flour - 4 tsp;
- egg - 2 pcs.;
- zucchini - 3 pcs.;
- olive oil for frying - 4 tbsp.;
- salt to taste.

Cooking method:

1. Peel the zucchini, grate, let the excess juice drain.
2. Add eggs, salt, coconut flour, if desired - grated cheese, chopped garlic and herbs.
3. Let the dough stand for 10 minutes.
4. Fry the pancakes in butter on each side.

# Carbohydrate-free diet

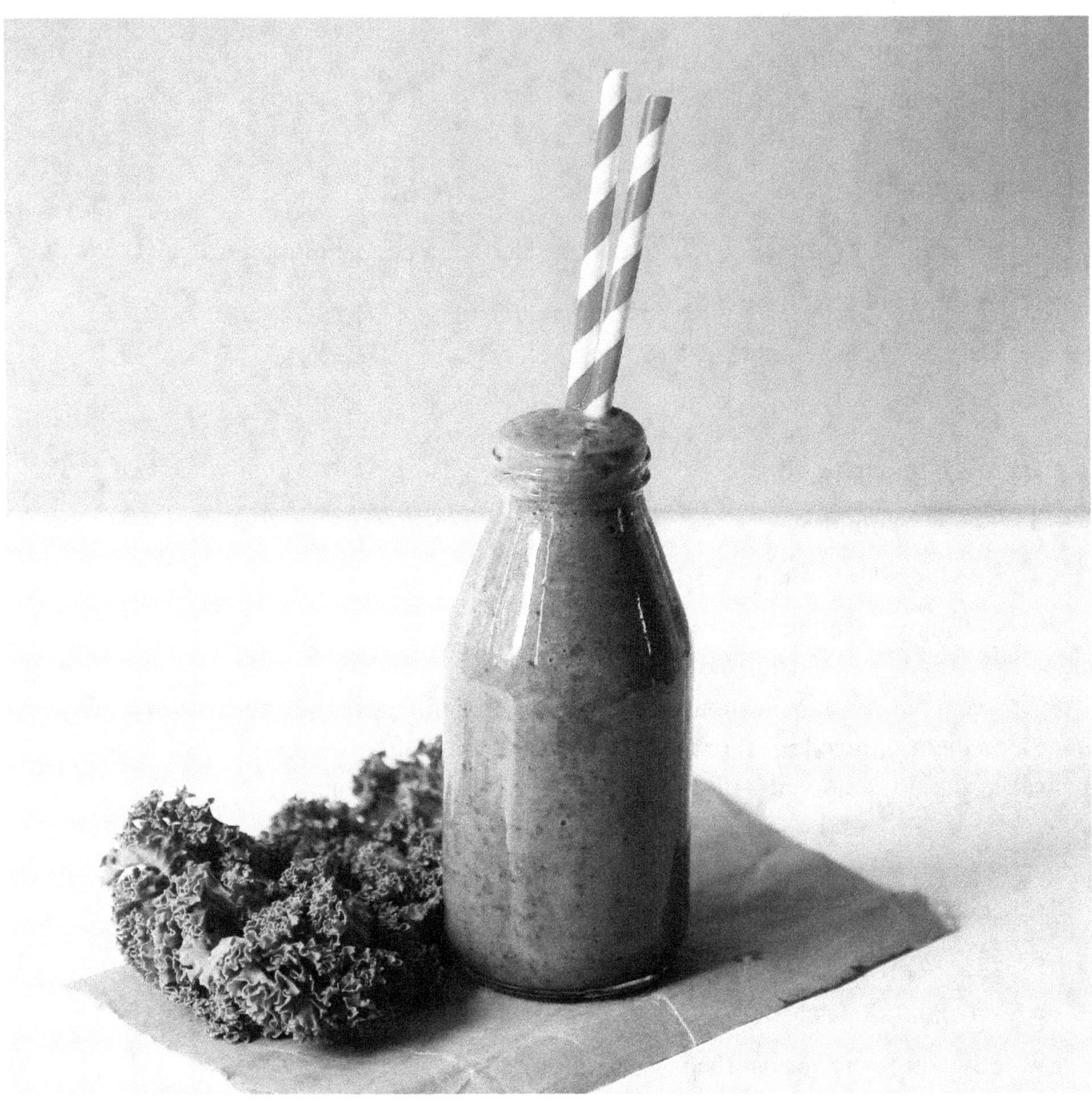

**Carbohydrate-Free Diet: A Weight Loss Menu**

Rapid weight loss is possible with a diet based on the use of low-carb foods. Thanks to nutritional schemes, the body enters a state of ketosis - it breaks down and processes its own fat cells. The advantage of the diet is that you do not have to feel hungry or exhaust yourself with physical activity.

**What is a Carbohydrate-Free Diet**

A low-carb diet is also called a high-fat diet, according to Atkins, or the keto diet. Losing weight according to this technique occurs due to changes in metabolic processes. The body needs glucose to nourish the tissues of the brain and internal organs. Most of this substance is obtained by a person by eating carbohydrates. Part of the glucose is used to feed all body systems, and its remnants are deposited under the skin in the form of glycogen - adipose tissue.

If a person goes on a low-carb diet, it may become glucose-deficient. To get the necessary substance, the body will begin to spend its reserves - to burn subcutaneous fat, extracting energy from it. As a result, the liver receives fatty acids, which are converted into ketone bodies through a long biochemical process. The process of ketosis is the basis for drying muscles for men and women athletes - marathon runners, triathletes, jocks.

**Efficiency**

Do not confuse ketosis with ketoacidosis (an extremely dangerous metabolic disorder). The process of converting fats into ketone bodies is not only safe, but, according to some doctors, helps in the treatment of Alzheimer's disease, reduces the number of seizures in patients with epilepsy and the risk of developing cancer. A carbohydrate-free diet is recommended as a therapeutic one in the presence of such indications:

- insulin resistance - tissue immunity to glucose;
- obesity;
- hypertension - a disease of the cardiovascular system, characterized by high blood pressure;
- polycystic ovary disease is a gynecological disease that occurs due to metabolic disorders.

**Stages of the Diet**

The process of ketosis does not start immediately. In order to go into a state of burning subcutaneous fat, the body needs to feel the lack of carbohydrates and analyze further actions. The developers of the keto diet claim that in order to lose weight, the body must go through 4 main stages of adaptation:

- Stage 1. The last time you eat carbs is breakfast. Devote lunch and dinner to carbohydrate-free foods. The supply of glucose obtained will dry up after 4-5 hours, after which the body will begin to process glycogen.
- Stage 2. On the 2-3rd day, the body realizes that there will be no more

carbohydrates and will begin to spend more reserves of alternative energy. The process of fat burning begins.

- Stage 3. It comes in 4-5 days, when almost all glycogen stores are exhausted. Subcutaneous fat is slowly melting, but the body has not yet entered the stage of ketosis and uses proteins to provide internal organs with energy. The third stage is associated with the rule of the ketosis diet: the need to increase the amount of protein foods during the first week.
- Stage 4. After a week, the process of ketosis starts at full strength, the body begins to actively burn subcutaneous fat.

## Rules and principles of nutrition

Do not expect a quick effect and do not try to speed up weight loss by starting to starve - eat often, but in small portions. In order not to harm yourself, you need to take into account the following nuances:

- Do not avoid proteins and unsaturated fats. Thanks to this combination of nutrients, the body compensates for carbohydrate starvation and provides adequate nutrition for the brain and soft tissues of internal organs. The required amount of protein can be calculated from the considerations that 1 g of protein should be supplied per 1 kg of weight. For example, your body weight is 85 kg, which means that you need to consume 85 g of protein compounds per day. Fat should be 3-4 times more.
- To maintain water-salt balance, drink plenty of fluids - at least 2 liters of water per day.
- Reduce the calorie content of your usual daily diet by 20%. Do not completely eliminate carbohydrates, but only reduce their amount to a minimum. Choose foods that contain complex organic compounds.
- You cannot be on a rigid carbohydrate-free weight loss scheme for more than 2 weeks. Even if you are very impressed with the first results, and there are no complaints about overall health, take a break for 4-5 months.

## How many carbohydrates should you eat on a carbohydrate-free diet

The keto nutrition system is divided into two types, depending on the amount of carbohydrates in the daily diet. These include:

- low-carb option. The menu assumes that in the first week you will consume no more than 40 g of carbohydrates per day, and starting from day 8, increase the amount of these organic compounds to 120 g.
- Protein-free option. You completely abandon all high-carbohydrate foods, reducing the daily amount of carbohydrates to 20 g.

## Carbohydrate-free diet for weight loss

Depending on the carbohydrate content and the need for training, all keto diets can also be divided into several other types. The most popular types of carbohydrate-free diets include:

- Constant diet. It implies a complete rejection of carbohydrates or their reduction to 20 grams per day, while organic matter must enter the body in the form of fiber. In a carbohydrate-free menu, the deficiency is compensated by a large amount of fat and protein. Thanks to a dietary scheme, you can get rid of 10-15 kg in a month, but you cannot constantly observe it due to the high risk of developing ketoacidosis.
- Power option. Suitable for those who combine weight loss with intense physical activity. In this case, carbohydrates should be consumed immediately before training in order to replenish glucose reserves. To increase performance, keto athletes are encouraged to take creatine monohydrate supplements.
- Cyclic nutrition pattern. Its essence is to consume only carbohydrate-free foods for the first 6 days (with the exception of the standard dose of 40 g). On the 7th day, it is recommended to return to good nutrition in order to saturate the muscles with glycogen and prevent the appearance of side effects - weakness, dizziness, decreased performance.

## What foods are allowed on the diet

The basis of a low-carb diet is the proteins found in meat, dairy products and eggs. You should also not deny yourself the use of oily fish, rich in omega-3 acids. Table of permitted foods and calorie content per 100 g:

|  | Calories, kcal | Amount of proteins, in grams | Amount of carbohydrates, in grams | Amount of fats, in grams |
|---|---|---|---|---|
| Vegetables and spices: | | | | |
| radish | 19 | 1.2 | 3.4 | 0.1 |
| cabbage | 27 | 1.8 | 4,7 | 0.1 |
| eggplant | 24 | 1.2 | 4.5 | 0.1 |
| broccoli | 28 | 3 | 5.2 | 0.4 |
| parsnip | 47 | 1.4 | 9.2 | 0.5 |
| basil | 27 | 2.5 | 4.3 | 0.6 |
| asparagus | 20 | 2 | 3.1 | 0.1 |
| cucumbers | 15 | 0.8 | 2.8 | 0.1 |
| legumes (lentils, peas) | 284 | 24 | 42.7 | 1.5 |
| tomatoes | 20 | 0.6 | 4.2 | 0.2 |
| Fruit: | | | | |
| avocado | 208 | 2 | 7, 4 | 20 |
| oranges | 36 | 1 | 8.1 | 0.2 |
| peaches | 46 | 1 | 11.3 | 0.1 |
| grapefruit | 29 | 0.7 | 6.5 | 0.2 |
| apples | 47 | 0.4 | 10 | 0.4 |
| Nuts: | | | | |
| almonds | 645 | 18.6 | 16.2 | 57.7 |
| coconuts | 354 | 3.4 | 6.2 | 33.5 |
| pistachios | 557 | 20.1 | 7 | 50 |
| Cereals and cereals: | | | | |
| buckwheat | 132 | 4.5 | 25 | 2.3 |
| quinoa | 367 | 14.1 | 57.3 | 6.1 |
| Dairy products: | | | | |
| parmesan | 392 | 33 | 0 | 28 |
| buttermilk 1% | 40 | 2.8 | 4 | 1 |
| yogurt 2% | 60 | 4.3 | 6.2 | 2 |
| Russian cheese | 363 | 24.1 | 0.3 | 29.5 |
| low-fat cottage cheese | 71 | 16.5 | 1.3 | 0 |
| skim milk | 31 | 2 | 4.8 | 0.1 |
| Meat: | | | | |
| beef | 187 | 19 | - | 19.4 |
| pork | 259 | 16 | - | 21.6 |
| lamb | 209 | 15.6 | - | 16.3 |
| bacon | 500 | 23 | - | 45 |
| ham | 279 | 22.6 | - | 21 |
| chicken | 190 | 16 | - | 14 |

| | | | | |
|---|---|---|---|---|
| Seafood and fish: | | | | |
| boiled shrimp | 95 | 19 | - | 2.2 |
| salmon | 142 | 20 | - | 6.3 |
| trout | 97 | 19.2 | - | 2.1 |
| Eggs: | | | | |
| fried eggs | 215 | 12 | 0.7 | 17.3 |
| boiled | 157 | 12 , 7 | 0.7 | 11 |

## What to exclude from the diet

Sweet desserts, fast food, starchy vegetables should be completely excluded from the menu. It is also worth avoiding those products that have undergone technical processing: freezing, conservation, pickling. They contain harmful preservatives, trans fats, and starch. As for natural sweeteners, they are also not welcome on a carbohydrate-free menu. In moderation, you can use natural sweeteners like stevia, agave syrup, honey, and sweet root vegetables (such as Jerusalem artichoke). A complete list of what to exclude from the diet:

| | Calories, kcal | Protein content Protein | content Carbohydrates | Fat content |
|---|---|---|---|---|
| Vegetables: | | | | |
| carrots | 32 | 1.3 | 6.9 | 0.1 |
| corn | 101 | 3.5 | 15.6 | 2.8 |
| Fruit: | | | | |
| bananas | 95 | 1, 5 | 22 | 0.2 |
| melon | 33 | 0.6 | 7.4 | 0.3 |
| figs | 49 | 0.7 | 13.7 | 0.2 |
| persimmons | 66 | 0.5 | 15.3 | 0.3 |
| Porridge: | | | | |
| semolina | 98 | 3 | 15.3 | 3.2 |
| white rice | 344 | 6.7 | 79 | 0.7 |
| Flour products: | | | | |
| pasta | 337 | 10.4 | 69.7 | 1.1 |
| dumplings | 155 | 7.6 | 18.7 | 2.3 |
| dumplings | 275 | 12 | 29 | 12.4 |
| wheat bread | 242 | 8.1 | 48.8 | 1 |
| Sweets: | | | | |
| sugar | 398 | - | 100 | - |
| curd mass with fruits or raisins | 343 | 6.8 | 29.9 | 21.6 |
| sweets | 456 | 4.3 | 67.5 | 20 |

## Drinks and alcohol

On a carbohydrate-free weight loss pattern, it is prohibited to abuse alcoholic beverages, beer, energy cocktails, and sweet soda. Preference should be given to mineral water without gas or the following liquids:

- rosehip decoction;
- linden or chamomile tea;
- green tea;
- coffee without sugar (no more than 1 time per day);
- tea with milk;
- natural sour fruit juices.

## Carb-free diet menu for the week

Once you understand the principles of low-carb diet, you can easily think about your diet for several days in advance. You can choose and combine any products from the list of allowed as you see fit. The main thing is not to exceed the norm of carbohydrates in 40 g. Approximate menu for 5 days:

|  | **Breakfast** | **Snack** | **Lunch** | **Snack** | **Dinner** |
|---|---|---|---|---|---|
| **Day 1** | Tea, a portion (200 g) of boiled brown rice, a glass of low-fat fermented baked milk | Cabbage salad with cucumbers, 3 walnuts. | Vegetable salad (300 g), chopped chicken cutlets - 200 grams. | Protein omelet (100 g) with a slice of cheese. | Fried flounder - 200 grams, 100 natural fat-free yogurt, 1 apple. |
| **Day 2** | Half a grapefruit. | Fried eggs from 2 eggs, green tea. | Boiled turkey fillet - 150-200 grams, any vegetable snack - 200 grams. | Rosehip broth, orange. | Seafood salad - 150 grams, salmon fillet baked in herbs - 200 grams. |
| **Day 3** | Curd casserole - 100 grams, tea. | 2 boiled eggs, a glass of low-fat fermented baked milk. | Beefsteak - 200 grams, stewed zucchini with cabbage - 150 g. | 2 slices of cheese, a glass of yogurt. | Flounder with grilled vegetables - 400 g. |
| **Day 4** | Protein omelet - 100 g, 2 slices of ham, rosehip broth. | 100 grams of yogurt, apple. | 200 grams of hake, stewed vegetables (zucchini, tomatoes, asparagus) - 100 g. | 100 grams of yogurt, apple. | 200 grams of beef, 100 grams of asparagus. |
| **Day 5** | Two-hundred-gram portion of buckwheat porridge, coffee without sugar. | An Apple. | Lean soup (without potatoes) - 250 ml, 100 grams of boiled pork. | The vinaigrette. | A glass of buttermilk, a slice of cheese, any vegetables - 100 grams. |

**Keto Diet Recipes**

You can cook meals on a low-carb diet by any methods. It is allowed to fry with vegetable or olive oil, but carbohydrate-free recipes are considered the healthiest, where cooking, stewing, baking in the oven, or steaming are used. Salads should not be seasoned with mayonnaise or sour cream sauces, preference should be given to refined oils of the first pressing, lemon juice.

**Turkey fillet baked with herbs**

- Time: 1 hour 40 minutes.
- Servings Per Container: 4 Persons.
- Calorie content: 134.6 kcal.
- Purpose: lunch or dinner.
- Cuisine: international.
- Difficulty: easy.

Delicious turkey meat is present in many dietary and medical tables. Fillet baked in herbs cooks very quickly. All you need to do is marinate the meat with spices in advance, put the dish in the oven. From spices to turkey fillet, rosemary, garlic, thyme, dry or fresh sage, black pepper are ideal.

Ingredients:

- turkey fillet - 1 kg;
- spices - 2 tbsp. l.;
- olive oil - 2 tbsp. l

Cooking method:

1. Peel the fillet from films, fat, rinse under running water.
2. Toss the spices separately with the salt and olive oil.
3. Rub each fillet generously with the marinade.
4. Leave to marinate for at least 20 minutes.
5. Preheat the oven to 200 ° C.
6. Place the fillets on a baking sheet lined with baking paper.
7. After 20 minutes, lower the oven temperature to 150 ° C, place the bird in it.
8. Bake the fillets for about an hour.
9. Then take the meat out of the oven, wrap it with foil.

10. Leave it on for 10 minutes. During this time, the fillet will reach readiness, but will not lose its juiciness.

**Grilled mackerel in foil**

- Time: 30 minutes.
- Servings Per Container: 3 Persons.
- Calorie content: 240 kcal.
- Purpose: dinner.
- Cuisine: international.
- Difficulty: easy.

Mackerel is a storehouse of minerals, vitamins and omega-2 fatty acids. It contains a lot of magnesium, potassium, sodium, sulfur, phosphorus, vitamins of groups A, B, D. Grilled, this fish turns out to be especially aromatic and juicy. You can please yourself and your loved ones with delicious fish both outdoors and at home, baking mackerel in the oven on the grill mode.

Ingredients:

- mackerel - 3 pcs .;
- lemon - 0.5 pcs.;
- parsley - 1 bunch.

Cooking method:

1. Wash well, gut the mackerel. Cut in half along the ridge (bones do not need to be removed).
2. Sprinkle pieces of fish with lemon juice, salt, season with parsley sprigs.
3. Wrap each piece tightly with foil.
4. Fry the fish over hot coals for about 7 minutes on each side, or grill in the oven for 10-15 minutes.

**Vegetable salad with seafood**

- Time: 25 minutes.
- Servings Per Container: 2 Persons.
- Calorie content: 147 kcal.
- Purpose: for breakfast, lunch, dinner.

- Cuisine: international.
- Difficulty: easy.

The classic combination of seafood and citrus fruits will appeal to everyone - both those who adhere to the rules of a carbohydrate-free method for losing weight, and simply connoisseurs of proper and tasty food. Such a salad is prepared very quickly. While the seafood is boiling, you can quickly chop up other ingredients. Greek yogurt is used for dressing.

Ingredients:

- shrimp - 150 g;
- grapefruit - 150 g;
- tomatoes - 2 pcs.;
- arugula - 100 g;
- avocado -1 half.

Cooking method:

1. Peel the shrimp from the shell and intestines.
2. Fry in butter for 2 minutes on each side.
3. Cut the avocado and tomatoes into small slices.
4. Place the washed and dried arugula on a dish.
5. Arrange the avocado on the sides of the plate, alternating with the tomatoes.
6. Gently place the shrimp in the center, tails up.

## Chicken broth soup with green beans

- Time: 40 minutes.
- Servings Per Container: 4 Persons.
- Calorie content: 567 kcal.
- Purpose: lunch.
- Cuisine: international.
- Difficulty: easy.

First courses are the basis of any diet. It is important to cook not only healthy, but also a variety of soups,  beetroot so that they do not get bored. If you're on a carb-free diet, try the chicken broth with green beans option. There are only 10 grams of carbohydrates per 100 grams of this soup.

Ingredients:

- boneless chicken breast - 3 pcs .;
- carrots - 2 pcs.;
- chicken broth - 1.5 liters;
- coriander seeds - 1 tsp;
- green beans - 250 g;
- spinach - 50 g;
- garlic - 2 cloves.

Cooking method:

1. Put it to heat or cook chicken broth.
2. Peel the carrots. Cut into thin slices along with the chicken breast.
3. Wash and dry the beans. Cut off the ends. Divide the long pods into halves.
4. Fry the chicken and carrots in a tall skillet in oil (5 minutes).
5. Add beans to the meat. Simmer, stirring occasionally, for 8 minutes.
6. Pour in the hot broth. Add chopped coriander seeds, boil for 10 minutes.
7. Place spinach and chopped garlic in a saucepan 2-3 minutes before the end of cooking.

**What to do in case of a breakdown**

The carbohydrate-free diet is rich and satisfying, but even with it there is a chance to break loose and go beyond the daily intake of carbohydrates. First, find out the cause of the breakdown and try to fix it. If you can't follow the rules clearly, look for another diet option. Otherwise, just keep following the principles.

**Exit from a carbohydrate-free diet**

When completing the course of a diet, try to start eating right so that the lost pounds do not return in excess. Try to stick to a low-carb menu. Remember that cereals, starchy vegetables should be eaten in the morning, and food without carbohydrates is for lunch and dinner. Observe the limitation of carbohydrates, increasing their consumption to 200 g per day.

**Contraindications**

A carbohydrate-free diet is not for everyone. During a diet, dizziness often appears, sensitivity to stressful situations, convulsions, and insomnia increases. It is strongly discouraged to follow the keto diet for children and adults in the presence of:

- pregnancy;
- diseases of the liver, kidneys;
- type 1 diabetes mellitus;
- serious diseases of the heart, vascular system;
- stomach diseases - colitis, ulcers;
- avitaminosis.

**Advantages and disadvantages of a carbohydrate-free menu**

A diet with a small amount of carbohydrates leads to a decrease in tissue resistance to insulin, helps to get rid of abdominal fat (on the abdomen, waist, hips). In addition, carbohydrate-free food "is able" to:

- increase the level of good cholesterol in the blood - normalizes the level of high density lipoproteins;
- lower blood pressure, normalize glucose levels;
- slow down the production of the hormone ghrelin, which is responsible for appetite and hunger;
- normalize metabolism.

A lot of benefits do not make keto nutrition universal. In some cases, long-term adherence to such a weight loss pattern can bring significant harm to the body:

- Due to the need for a limited intake of cereals and fiber, the body will not receive the necessary nutrients, which may simply not be in meat, eggs or fish.
- Heavy protein foods hinder the digestion process, can disrupt the work of the pancreas, and cause constipation.
- Lack of glucose will affect your overall well-being. Your working capacity, mental activity will significantly decrease, due to a lack of energy, active physical activity will be given more difficulty.
- Protein breakdown products can increase the risk of developing liver disease, urolithiasis, atherosclerosis, and exacerbation of gout.

# Moscow/Kremlin diet

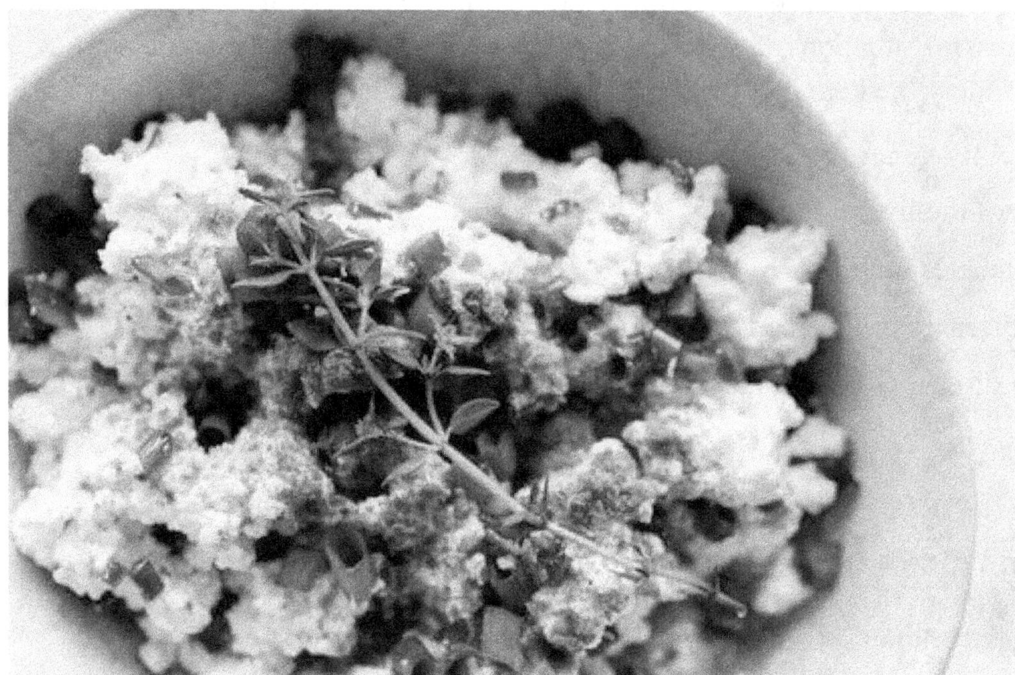

**Moscow diet: a table of products and menus for weight loss**

A popular Moscow diet, which is based on reducing carbohydrates, is considered the most effective and safe for the body. This technique is used by many famous artists, politicians. Sticking to a diet for only seven days, you can quickly lose up to 6 kg, and in 30 days this figure can be from 7 to 13 kg.

**Moscow diet for weight loss**

The Kremlin/Moscow weight loss technique was long considered as top secret. This diet includes foods with a low glycemic index. The mechanism of system action is similar to the Atkins diet - if there is no intake of carbohydrates, the body actively begins to process its own fat, which contributes to rapid weight loss.

For the convenience of losing weight by the Moscow diet, it was specially developed tables, with products and its symbols in points ( units) indicated. One point is a conventional unit, where 1 g of carbohydrates accounts for 100 g of the product. With the help of this table of the Moscow diet, you can easily plan your daily menu and choose suitable recipes. The technique allows the use of cheeses, meat and products containing a small amount of sugar.

**Principles and Effectiveness**

The essence of the Moscow method of losing weight is that it is necessary to drastically reduce the intake of carbohydrates. The body will begin to consume internal reserves of adipose tissue. This will make it possible for a short period of time to find the figure of your dreams. Scoring and calorie restrictions can be used to enhance the effectiveness of the diet. It is important not to eat 4 hours before bedtime. In order for the technique to give a positive result, speed up metabolism and not harm the body, it is necessary to adhere to the following basic principles:

- to avoid dehydration of the body, you should drink at least 1.5 liters of clean water;
- during the Kremlin method, sugar, potatoes, alcohol, flour products, rice are prohibited;
- in the first week it is necessary to limit the consumption of fruits and vegetables;
- you cannot starve, because this will have a negative effect on the losing weight;
- it is necessary in the first week 3 days to "eat" 40 points, then go to 20;
- vitamins and minerals should be added to the diet.


**Table of products**

The Moscow method of losing weight involves the use of a special table in points (1 point = 1 g of carbohydrates). The value of certain foods, for example, meat, is zero, but this does not mean that any food can be eaten in unlimited quantities. If you need to quickly get rid of several kilograms, then in the first 7 days you should limit yourself to 20 points per day, then during the second and third weeks - 30. During the consolidation of the result, you can eat foods daily, which in total should not be more than 40 points. Approximate table of the Kremlin diet:

| Products | Quantity in grams | Points |
|---|---|---|
| White bread | 100 | 48 |
| Boiled meat | 100 | 0 |
| Semolina | 150 | 40 |
| Sausages | 100 | 1 |
| Eggs | 60 | 0.5 |
| Sausage | 100 | 1 |
| Milk | 250 | 6 |
| Sour cream | 200 | 10 |
| buttermilk | 250 | 13 |
| Ham | 100 | 1 |
| Fried potatoes | 100 | 20 |
| Cabbage fresh | 100 | 5 |
| Mushrooms | 100 | 6 |
| Butter | 20 | 1 |
| Green pepper | 100 | 9 |
| Pasta | 250 | 32 |
| Pea soup | 500 | 20 |
| Maize | 100 | 15 |
| Chocolate cake | 150 | 70 |

## Kremlin diet menu

The diet of the Moscow method of losing weight consists primarily of protein foods. With this method, any meat is allowed: beef, pork, poultry, veal, as well as sausages, sausages, bacon, bacon. At the same time, against the background of an abundance of protein products, it is necessary to radically limit carbohydrate foods. If the body does not receive carbohydrates from foods, then it will begin to expand fat reserves accumulated over the years.

During the first two weeks of the Moscow system, plant food should be completely excluded, because it contains a lot of carbohydrates. During this period, sugar, cereals and sweets should be removed from the diet. The basis of the menu should be: cheese, meat, seafood, cottage cheese, fish, eggs. In addition, the use of certain alcoholic beverages is not prohibited: vodka, beer, cognac, brandy.

## Diet for three days

If you follow the strict recommendations of the Kremlin diet, you can easily get rid of 5 kg in a few days. This figure can grow up to 13 kg per month. To achieve the greatest effect, you need to monitor your carbohydrate intake and calorie intake. At the same time, nutritionists do not advise eating 4 hours before bedtime. For people who do not want to eat meat products for a long time, an express diet for 3 days is suitable:

| Days | Breakfast | Lunch | Afternoon snack | Dinner |
|---|---|---|---|---|
| 1 | Fried eggs from three eggs, tea without sugar, 100 g of cheese | Vegetable salad, celery soup, steak | 50 g of walnuts | 200 g boiled chicken, tomato |
| 2 | Tea without sugar, 2 boiled eggs, cottage cheese | Vegetable salad with butter, cabbage soup with sour cream, shish kebab | 200 g cheese | Fried chicken breast, boiled cauliflower |
| 3 | 100 g fried eggplant, 3 boiled sausages, tea without sugar | Cheese soup with vegetables, cabbage salad, pork chop | 10 olives | Boiled fish, tomato, a glass of buttermilk |

## Diet for a week

The approximate menu of the Kremlin method for 7 days is given as an example, so that it is easier for those who are losing weight to navigate and make their own. For personal taste, dishes can be added or reversed. The main condition is the use of 20 points per day in the first week, 30 points in the second and third weeks.

### Approximate diet for a week:

| Days of the week | Breakfast | Lunch | Afternoon snack | Dinner |
|---|---|---|---|---|
| Monday | Cottage cheese, 2 eggs with mushrooms, tea | Soup with meat, 100 g of fresh vegetables, unsweetened coffee | Hard cheese | Whole tomato, fried chicken, tea |
| Tuesday | 4 boiled sausages, fresh cauliflower, sugar-free coffee | 150 g vegetables, lamb skewers, sugar-free tea | Walnuts | 200 g lettuce, fried fish |
| Wednesday | 2 eggs, cheese, sugar-free coffee | 100 g boiled squid, baked mushrooms, sugar-free tea | 10 black olives | 200 g boiled fish , tomato, any fermented milk product |
| Thursday | 2 fried eggs, a cup of green tea | Boiled fish, low-fat pork chop | Orange | Baked chicken breast with cheese, 100 g of lettuce |
| Friday | 3 boiled eggs, cheese, coffee without sugar | Escalope, 100 g of fresh grated carrots with mayonnaise | 30 g of peanuts | Hard cheese, 150 ml of red wine, lettuce leaves |
| Saturday | Unsweetened tea, 200 g of cottage cheese with greens | Fish soup, 150 g of grated beets | 50 g of pumpkin seeds | 200 g of any boiled fish, lettuce leaves |
| Sunday | 150 g of cab caviar, 4 boiled sausages, | Cucumber salad, fried pork loin, tea without sugar | Any berry, mineral water | 200 g of lettuce leaves, a piece of fried fish |

## Diet for 14 days

The menu of the Moscow protein diet for 2 weeks is approximate, so portions and dishes can be swapped , replacing them with similar products in terms of the amount of carbohydrates. The main thing is that it is necessary to count according to the table, and then in half a month you can reduce the weight by 6 kilograms. An approximate menu of the Kremlin's weight loss method for 14 days:

| Days of the week | Breakfast | Lunch | Afternoon snack | Dinner |
|---|---|---|---|---|
| Monday | Cottage cheese, 2 chicken eggs, green tea | Borsch with meat, vegetable salad, | 200 g of hard cheese | Tomato, fried chicken, tea |
| Tuesday | 100 g of fresh cauliflower, 4 boiled sausages, tea | Vegetables with mushrooms, fried lamb, water | 5 almond kernels, a glass of mineral water | Vegetable salad, a piece of fried fish, tea |
| Wednesday | 150 g cheese, 2 eggs, green tea | Seafood salad with olives, a piece of fish with mushrooms | Olives | Yogurt, tomato , boiled fish |
| Thursday | Tea, omelet of three eggs with brisket | 200 g boiled squid, pork, sugar-free coffee | Apple | Lettuce, baked chicken breast with cheese, tea |
| Friday | 4 fried eggs, compote | 100 g raw carrots, escalope | 50 g peanuts | Light salad , a glass of red wine, 200 g of boiled fish |
| Saturday | Coffee without sugar, 150 g of cottage cheese | Salad with fresh beets, ear | 60 g of pumpkin seeds | Lettuce leaves, chicken fillet |
| Sunday | 4 sausages, caviar from zucchini | 200 g of boiled meat, salad with cucumber, tea | Olives | 150 g of fried fish, lettuce leaves, tea |

Starting from the 8th day, the menu can be repeated from the beginning or the food can be changed, while observing the main condition - to eat no more than 30 g of carbohydrates per day.

## Exit from the diet

The Moscow method of losing weight, based on the carbohydrate table of foods, is easy to follow, because losing weight does not experience hunger. To get out of the diet, you should gradually add 10 g of carbohydrates to the diet, so that the daily rate of 120 g is approximately obtained. It is important to ensure that the menu contains not simple, but complex carbohydrates (cereals, vegetables, legumes). It is necessary to maintain the absence of carbohydrate dependence as long as possible. In the future, you should control the amount of calories and do not forget to count them.

## Contraindications

Severe restriction of carbohydrates leads to weight loss, but this technique is not suitable for all people. The glucose found in sweet foods is essential for the body because it is a source of energy. Its deficiency can lead to decreased physical activity and weakened mental performance. Before starting to use the Moscow diet, you should definitely consult your doctor. You can not use the technique for lactating and pregnant women, elderly people and young people. Nutritionists advise against using the Kremlin diet in the presence of:

- diabetes;
- cardiovascular disease;
- kidney disease;
- alimentary violations;
- diseases of the gastrointestinal tract;
- depression and nervous lability.

# Cleansing diets

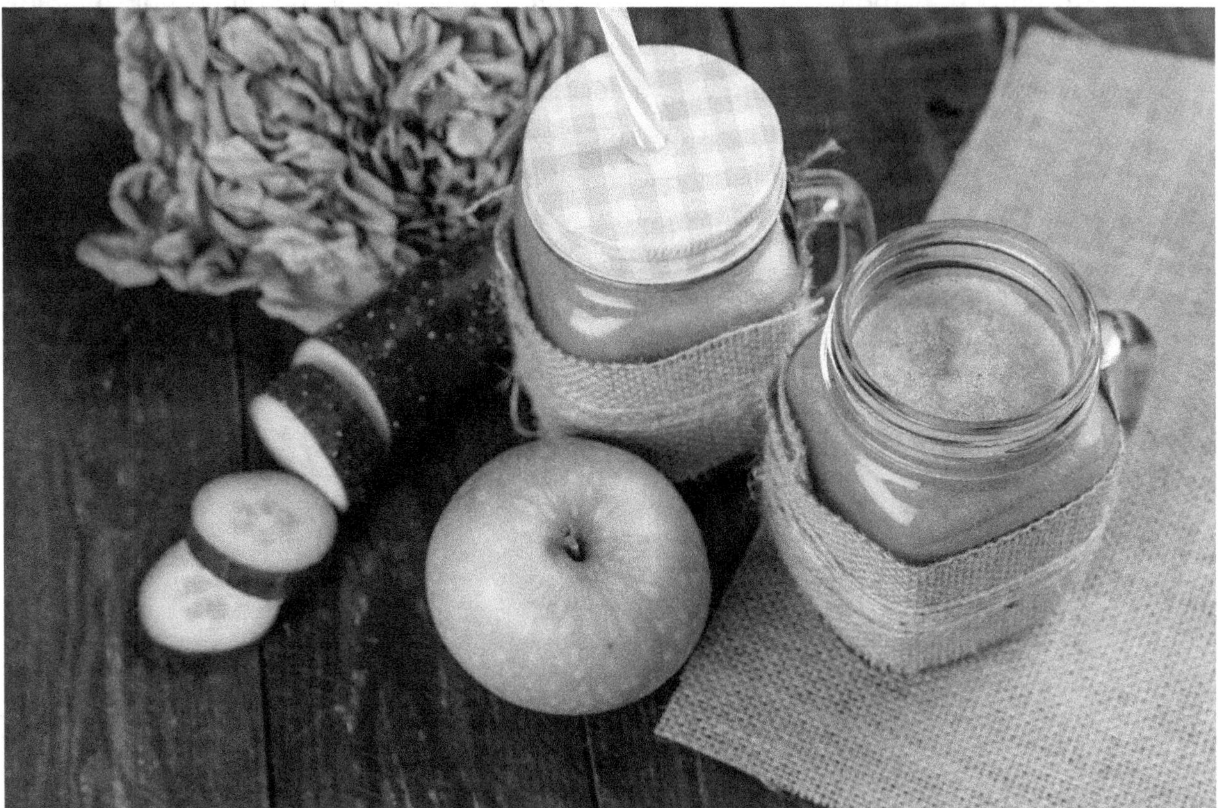

Specialized nutrition in 60% of cases helps to get rid of slagging of the body. There are diets based on products that remove toxins and neutralize poisons. Cleansing systems include the following nutritional systems: detox, pectin, fiber, diuretic, porridge. It must be observed strictly according to the rules.

**What is a cleansing diet**

Under the definition of cleansing diets are nutritional systems for removing toxins from the body. Observing them, you need to adhere to the following rules and principles:

Get a medical examination before introducing changes in the diet. Permission must be given by a doctor or nutritionist. The categorical contraindications are oncology, genetic pathologies, pregnancy and lactation, epilepsy, exacerbations of chronic diseases, mental disorders.

A few weeks before starting a diet, try to switch to proper nutrition. Do not overuse harmful products. Introduce fiber-rich foods in your diet. Follow your drinking regimen. The rate of consumed water per day is 30 ml / 1 kg of body weight. Add another 1-2 glasses to the resulting value.

Food to cleanse the body should be fractional. Eat small meals every 3-4 hours. After eating, it is advisable to avoid excessive physical activity for half an hour.

Don't eat too late. The last meal is 4 hours before bedtime.

Prepare fresh meals for 1 day.

Chew food vigorously. Don't drink it down. Drinks are allowed to be consumed either half an hour before meals, or after.

If you feel unwell, return to your standard diet. After a while, try another cleansing food system.

# Metabolic diet

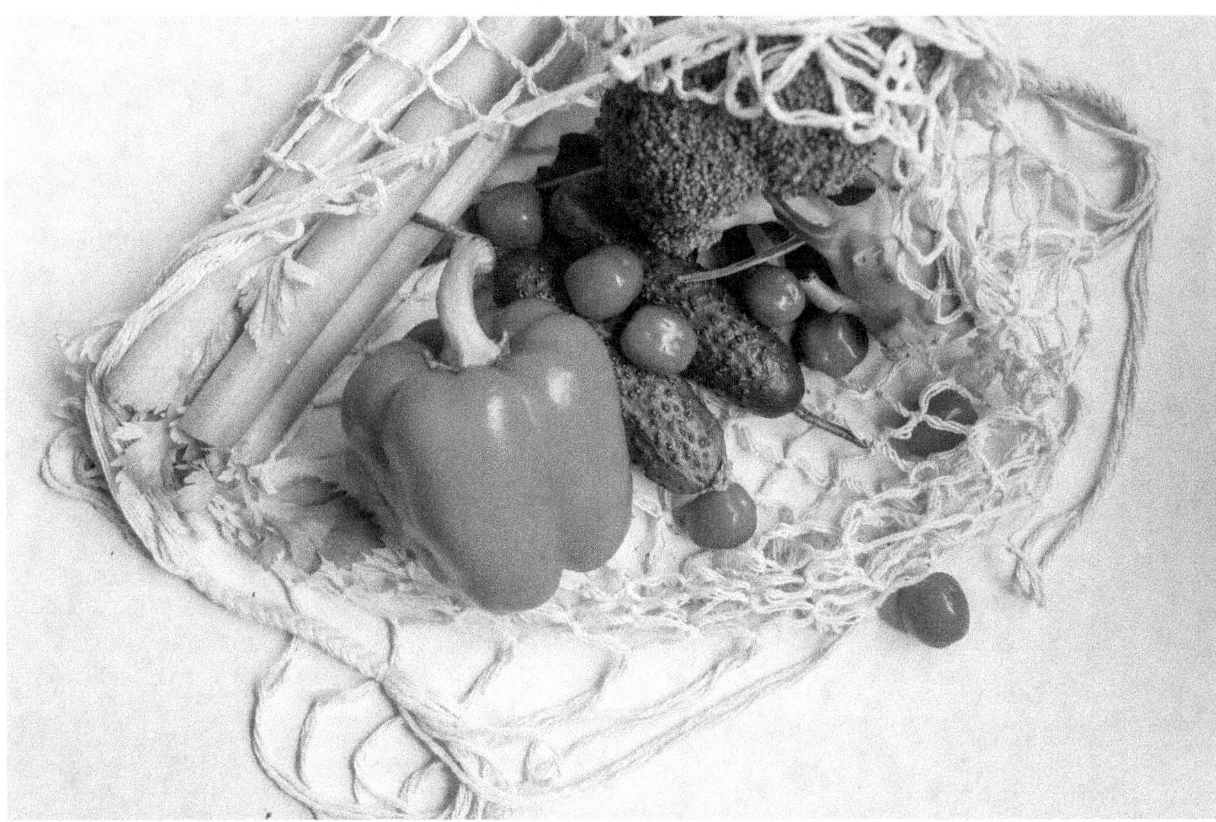

**Metabolic diet - an everyday menu**

This system is one of the most effective and efficient - it helps to lose excess body fat by accelerating metabolic processes in the body. The metabolic diet is not harmful to health, but it is recommended to follow it for a long time. The result will surely please everyone who is losing weight - the monthly weight loss will be 2-6 kg, which is unlikely to return back to your body.

**What is a metabolic diet**

The essence of the diet is to stabilize hormonal levels, normalize metabolic processes, and cleanse the body of toxins. The system menu is designed so that the production of some hormones is inhibited, while others, on the contrary, are accelerated. Estrogen and insulin, which contribute to the accumulation of fat stores, will be synthesized more slowly. Testosterone and adrenaline will be produced in greater quantities - just their action is aimed at burning fat. The normalized hormonal balance of the body allows you to lose weight and prevent it from being reset.

When following a diet, it is important to hand out food correctly throughout the day. At breakfast, you need to eat a complex of carbohydrates. The calorie content of the menu for every day is calculated by points - after waking up there should be more of them, and, starting with lunch, the indicator gradually decreases. During the evening meal, it is permissible to eat only protein foods and vegetables.

A metabolic diet can only be observed for people who do not have health problems; it is also practiced with metabolic syndrome - this is a symptom complex of metabolic disorders that arise against the background of obesity and are caused by disorders of carbohydrate metabolism. The disease is not a medical diagnosis, but statistics prove that about 2.5 million people on the planet suffer from it. The metabolic syndrome is expressed mainly in obesity, but its presence is also evidenced by other signs:

- increased drowsiness after eating protein foods;
- constant feeling of thirst;
- the appearance of weakness if you cannot take food on time;
- increased sweating during night sleep;
- feeling of hunger is accompanied by apathy or increased aggression;
- there is always a desire to eat at least some kind of sweetness, a person is tormented by attacks of rapid heartbeat.

## Pros and Cons

Reviews of the metabolic diet confirm that this is one of the easiest, but effective weight loss systems - there is no need to force your body with hunger strikes or strain, counting calories every day. In addition, it has an amount of other advantages:

- Balanced, easy to carry. The diet can be followed for a long time, changing your eating habits - thanks to the normalization of nutrition, on average, you can lose weight by 3-5 kg per month.
- Metabolism improves, the functions of the gastrointestinal tract, hormones are normalized.
- The skin becomes elastic, smooth.
- The menu for each day contains different products, so there is no feeling of hunger.
- If necessary, it is allowed to skip the first stage of the diet. Weight will still decrease, although not as quickly as if all consecutive phases are observed.

## As for the disadvantages:

- The menu of the first stage of the metabolic diet involves a sharp restriction of simple carbohydrates, which causes some difficulties with its further passage.

- In the first weeks, due to the restructuring of the body, unpleasant senses are observed in the form of increased flatulence in the intestines.

**General rules**

To speed up metabolism implies a competent distribution of food for each meal during the day, due to which metabolic processes are stabilized. The diet has a simple nutritional scheme, the menu is based on scoring. All foods have points based on their calorie content. Having switched to this diet, you must adhere to a number of rules:

- To create a menu for every day, you need to add points. It is important to avoid exceeding them in certain meals.
- You can not exceed the level of points, you can eat less.
- If you miss a meal, you cannot add points for lunch, dinner, or breakfast.
- Between meals, a maximum of 3 hours break is allowed.
- The volume of a single serving should not exceed 250 g.
- It is important to drink a glass of water on an empty stomach.
- Do not eat before bed - the last meal should take place 3 hours before rest.
- It is recommended to drink about 2 liters of water every day.
- When following a metabolic diet, it is advisable to take medications that provide the body with useful vitamins and minerals.
- Steaming and braising are acceptable methods of cooking food. Fried foods should be excluded.
- The amount of salt, seasonings, spices and semi-finished products consumed is recommended to be minimized or completely limited during the diet.
- It is advisable to give preference to plant foods (fruits, vegetables), cereals, cottage cheese and other fermented milk and dairy products and drinks.
- It is permissible to eat bread on a diet, but it must be made with bran or whole grain flour.
- You can eat meat once a day, but only if it belongs to dietary varieties. In other meals, it is allowed to replace it with chicken eggs or fish.
- The diet menu must include nuts, dried fruits, legumes, which help to strengthen the cardiovascular system.
- The norm of sugar for every day should not be more than 20 g.
- Any food should be eaten, chewing thoroughly.

## Main phases

The metabolic recovery diet consists of three phases, which must be followed in sequence. They consist in the following:

- The first stage - fat burning, lasting 10-14 days. Weight is reduced quickly, but it will be necessary to follow a rigid menu, in which the consumption of fats (up to 1 tablespoon of olive oil / day) and carbohydrate food is sharply limited. The stage cannot be observed for more than 2 weeks, while in case of deterioration in well-being, the time frame may be reduced. It is recommended to negotiate the specific terms of compliance with the first phase with a nutritionist, because they also depend on the characteristics of the body of a particular person. At the fat-burning stage, only meals with 0 points are allowed every day. The menu is dominated by protein products - low-fat dairy drinks and diet meats. The diet is allowed to be supplemented with fresh vegetables.

- The second phase is normalization, which lasts 14-90 days. This stage is the longest - it will last until the balance arrow shows the desired result. Fat is burned gradually, but steadily, which eliminates the occurrence of health problems. Each meal must have a certain number of points: breakfast - 4, 2nd breakfast - 2, lunch - 2, snack - 1, dinner - only zero.

- The third stage is consolidation. The duration of the last phase has no restrictions - you can eat, taking into account food points, every day for the rest of your life. The fixing phase is aimed at stabilizing the achieved result. Losing weight, it is most tolerated - by this time the body has time to fully adapt to the new dietary menu. The stage does not cause physiological or psychological discomfort, because the refusal of junk food has already become a habit. At the stage of consolidation, 1 point is added to each meal (except for dinner, it must contain 0 points).

## Metabolic Food Diet Table

The basis of the diet is a specially designed table. It is based on the selection of products, taking into account their carbohydrate value - from the lowest value to the highest. When compiling a dietary menu for every day, choose the ingredients from the list below, combine them with each other:

| 0 points | 1 point | 2 points | 3 points | 4 points |
|---|---|---|---|---|
| Any fresh vegetables<br>Rabbit meat<br>Mushrooms<br>All white poultry<br>Quail / chicken eggs<br>Low-fat fish, seafood, algae<br>Any fresh herbs<br>Garlic and onions<br>Green peas<br>Lemon, lime<br>Fiber, bran<br>Sour milk / milk drinks with a fat content of up to 2%<br>Sour apples<br>Spices, horseradish, mustard, apple and grape vinegar<br>Protein cocktails, bars | Fresh vegetables<br>White beans and other legumes<br>Any fresh berries | Boiled carrots, beets<br>Bran bread<br>Feta, feta cheese<br>Chicken<br>Veal<br>Lamb<br>Beef<br>Avocado<br>Dairy and sour milk products, the fat content of which does not exceed 4%<br>Oatmeal, buckwheat porridge<br>Any fresh nuts, seeds<br>Fruits<br>By-products<br>Unpeeled or wild rice<br>Olives, olives<br>Vegetable oil<br>Muesli | fruit slices<br>Fruit juices<br>Hard and processed cheeses<br>Bitter chocolate<br>Wheat groats<br>Corn<br>Whole grain muesli | Lean pork<br>Any sweets, incl. sugar, chocolate, condensed milk, honey<br>Semolina, pasta, mayonnaise<br>Baking and fresh bread<br>Dairy and fermented milk products with a fat content of more than 4%<br>Beer and other alcohol<br>Duck and goose<br>Juices from packages<br>Carbonated drinks, incl. lemonade<br>Chips<br>Canned food in oil, sausages, sausages, etc.<br>Dried fruits<br>Potatoes<br>Ice cream |

## How to calculate points correctly

In order for the metabolic diet menu to give the desired result, you need to learn how to eat on a point system every day. For example, if a meal should be 5 points, you can get this amount in several ways:

- Take 2 products out of 2 points, 1 - one point.
- Supplement a 4-point product with a product containing 1 point.
- Take a 3-point product and a 2-point product, if necessary, you can also add a zero one. It is recommended to choose food with a lower score, combine several different products.

## Everyday Menu

When deciding to switch to a metabolic weight loss system, some people face certain difficulties, for example, combining products according to a point table, making a suitable menu from them. This will help you overcome all difficulties and still get rid of excess weight. Find out what the metabolic diet menu should be for every day.

## Menu of the 1st phase of the metabolic diet

| Days of the week | Breakfast | 2nd breakfast | Lunch | Snack | Dinner |
|---|---|---|---|---|---|
| Monday | Omelet of 2 eggs with the addition of milk, salad (cucumber, tomato, olive oil) | Cottage cheese 0% fat, tea without sugar, but with lemon | Fish broth, stewed mushrooms, cucumber | Seaweed, salad of garlic and fresh carrots, seasoned with lemon juice | Boiled chicken fillet, salad of vegetables (bell pepper and tomatoes) |
| Tuesday | Oven-baked chicken fillet, green peas, unsweetened tea A | glass of low-fat milk, bran flour loaf | Minestrone soup, stewed rabbit meat, tomato and cucumber salad | Steamed cod, green peas | Stewed or baked turkey, steamed broccoli |
| Wednesday | Bran with dried fruit and a glass of milk | Hard boiled egg, a glass of low-fat buttermilk | Soup, green broccoli puree apple A | glass of milk with a fat content of 1-1.5% | Summer salad, a piece of boiled chicken fillet Fried |
| Thursday | eggs from 2 eggs | Protein bar | Roast rabbit with vegetables | 2 apples | Salad with green peas and onions, stewed mushrooms |
| Friday | Poached egg, natural yogurt | Glass of milk | Lean green borscht, boiled chicken fillet | Kiwi, orange | Vegetable stew, soft-boiled egg |
| Saturday | Mushroom casserole | Salad of 2-3 kinds of fruits | Mushroom julienne with chicken | glass of milk | Shrimp, grilled vegetables |
| Sunday | Egg poached | mousse berry | soup with pieces of fish | Grapefruit | Soy burgers, a salad of grated carrots |

## Second phase of the metabolic diet

| Days of the week | breakfast | 2nd breakfast | Lunch | Snack | Dinner |
|---|---|---|---|---|---|
| Monday | Whole Grain cereals | Bit of nuts | oatmeal with dried fruit | a glass of any berry | puree of eggplant, chicken roll |
| Tuesday | Salad from crab sticks with sweet corn, cucumber and greens, seasoned with sour cream | Bit of peanut | Buckwheat porridge with milk 1% fat | glass of carrot juice | Mushroom casserole, orange |
| Wednesday | Hard-boiled egg, orange juice | Bit of seeds | Meatless cabbage rolls | glass of tomato juice | Turkey steamed cutlets, baked zucchini |
| Thursday | Yoghurt with fresh fruit pieces, egg ruta A | glass of vegetable juice | Pilaf from unpeeled rice with any mushrooms | Green peas | Rabbit meat baked with vegetables |
| Friday | Processed cheese, a steam omelet of 2 eggs | Fresh vegetable Fresh | steamed beef cutlets, green peas | Chickpeas | Grilled fish with vegetables |
| Saturday | porridge Millet milk | Bit of walnuts | Pancakes liver Chicken | Berry mousse | salad shrimp and seaweed |
| Sunday | boiled egg, yogurt with fresh fruit | glass tomato juice | Meatball veal, bean puree | Bit of peanut | ragout vegetables boiled chicken |

## Third phase of the metabolic diet

The rules of the metabolic system imply that in the last phase, add 1 point to each meal. If the weight does not stand still, but continues to reduce, then after a week you can add 1 more point to all receptions, except for dinner. The total amount of points allowed in the menu of the third stage of the metabolic diet. It is determined individually for each person.Stabilization of weight at one point plays a decisive role here.

| Eating | Points Allowed |
|---|---|
| Breakfast | 5 |
| Second breakfast | 3 |
| Lunch | 3 |
| Snack | 2 |
| Dinner | 0 |

## Recipes

To make the metabolic diet as comfortable as possible for everyone, nutritionists have developed special recipes for delicious and easy-to-cook meals that have a certain amount of points. Consider the following examples to guide you on how to properly combine foods to get food on a point system.

### Salad with beans and chicken breast

Salad is one-point - it can be used with any approach to the table, except for dinner, starting with the second stage of the metabolic diet. It is allowed to add red or white beans, but before use it must be prepared - soak for 3-12 hours in water, then boil. Learn how to make a delicious, mouth-watering and easy salad with chicken breast and vegetables.

Ingredients:

- beans - 100 g;
- red onion - 1 pc .;
- lettuce leaves - 5 pcs.;
- cherry tomatoes - 2-4 pcs.;
- seasonings - to taste;
- chicken fillet - 0.5 kg;
- lemon juice - 1-2 tsp.

### Cooking method:

1. Wash the chicken fillet well, remove films and streaks. Boil until is ready, slightly salt the water. Chill meat completely, cut into small slices or tear with your hands.
2. Boil the beans. Chill completely.
3. Chop the onion into thin half rings.
4. Cut each tomato into 4 pieces.
5. Add meat, tomatoes, onion half rings, beans to the salad onionl. Sprinkle the ingredients with freshly squeezed lemon juice and stir.

**Casserole of green beans, eggs and greenery**

Such a two-point dish will become a satisfying meal for losing weight. You can replace the greens indicated in the recipe with any other and the amount also varies according to your taste preferences.

Ingredients:

- parsley, onion - 0.5 bunch each;
- vegetable oil (for refueling) - 1 tbsp. l .;
- egg - 1 pc .;
- green beans - 200 g;
- spinach - 0.5 bunch;
- seasonings, salt - to taste.

Cooking method:

1. Boil green beans: 8 minutes, put them in boiling water, frozen - pour cold water and cook for 8 minutes after the liquid boils.
2. Drain the excess water from the beans.
3. Wash the spinach and greens, cut into small pieces.
4. Mix both.
5. Add oil, salt to taste..
6. Put the workpiece in a fireproof mold, pour an egg beaten with a fork.
7. Bake the dish at 180 degrees for 20-25 minutes.

**Baked turkey cutlets with cheese**

Three-point dish - it can be eaten for breakfast in the second phase or made for almost any meal at the final stage of the diet. It is recommended to bake cutlets in the oven, while it is better to make minced meat, using fresh turkey fillets and spices. You can take any cheese, but it is better if it has a minimum fat content.

Ingredients:

- turkey fillet - 0.5 kg;
- hard cheese - 100 g;
- dill - 0.5 bunch;
- spices, salt - to taste.

Cooking method:

1. Use a blender to turn the fillet into minced meat. Add chopped herbs, spices to the mass, salt the workpiece.
2. Cut the hard cheese into small cubes, add to the meat mass.
3. Mix everything thoroughly, form small cutlets, put them in a fireproof dish, close it tightly with foil.
4. Bake the cutlets in an oven heated to 180 degrees. Serve the dish after 30-40 minutes.

# The Pectin diet

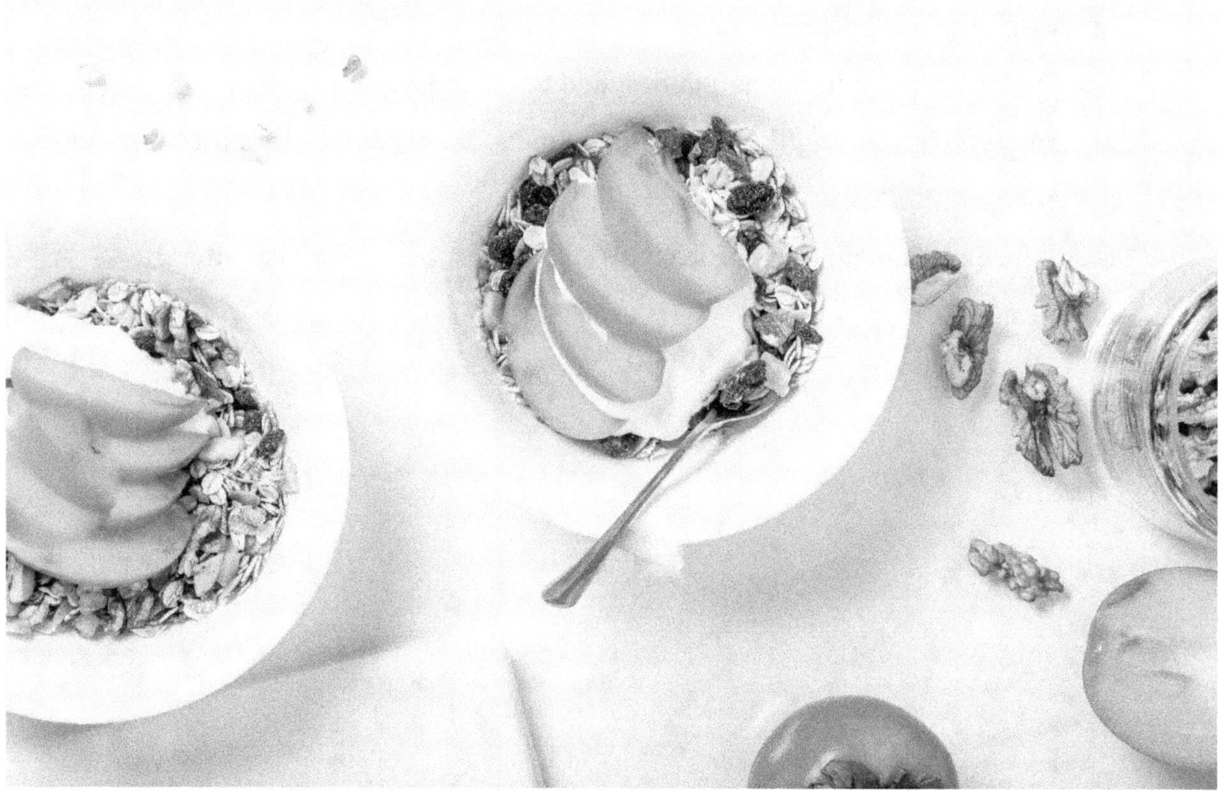

**Pectin Detox Diet**

This nutritional system is often prescribed to their patients for detoxification by nutritionists. Features:

1. The essence of the diet is to use foods rich with pectin. The substance removes slags, toxins, radionuclides and cholesterol from the body.

2. The pectin diet is indicated for slagging the body, digestive problems, overweight, high cholesterol levels.

3. The duration of the cleansing regime is a week. Experts do not recommend exceeding this period. This is fraught with vitamin deficiency due to the leaching of nutrients. Contraindications - stomach ulcer, pancreatitis, cholecystitis.

4. The more apples you eat, the more effective your diet will be.

## What the diet consists

The menu is made up according to the table:

| Allowed foods | Limited (you can eat no more than 1-2 times a week) | Forbidden |
|---|---|---|
| apricots;<br>eggs;<br>bananas;<br>apples of all varieties (fresh, baked, grated, juice);<br>beans;<br>citrus zest;<br>grapes;<br>pumpkin;<br>walnuts;<br>plums;<br>green tea;<br>beet;<br>lemons;<br>rice;<br>carrot;<br>peaches. | porridge;<br>lean fish;<br>milk products;<br>chicken breast. | alcoholic drinks;<br>chips and other snacks;<br>bakery products;<br>pears;<br>carbonated drinks;<br>melons;<br>sausages;<br>sweets;<br>confectionery;<br>vegetable oil;<br>coffee;<br>zucchini;<br>pasta;<br>potatoes;<br>ice cream;<br>radish;<br>squash;<br>meat. |

## Menu

Diet option for two days:

| Meal | First day | Second day |
|---|---|---|
| Breakfast | 150 g oatmeal with berries, 1 boiled egg. | 150 g of rice porridge in water, 2 slices of hard cheese. |
| Lunch | 200 ml of apple, berry, carrot smoothie. | 2 green apples. |
| Lunch | 150 g of stewed beans with herbs and grated carrots, 100 g of boiled chicken breast, 1 apple. | 150 g of buckwheat in water, 100 g of steamed sea fish, 1 peach. |
| Afternoon snack | 3-4 plums. | 150 g baked pumpkin. |
| Dinner | 200 g salad of low-fat cottage cheese, carrots, apples, seasoned with honey and lemon juice. | 150 g lentils, 150 g grated carrot and beetroot salad, 1 apple. |

# Cleansing fiber diet

The following diet is very beneficial and highly regarded by nutritionists. Features:

1. The basis of the diet is foods rich in dietary fiber. Fiber is not digested by enzymes and is excreted naturally. It improves digestion, restores intestinal microflora and cleanses from harmful substances. The fibers swell, giving a feeling of fullness for a long time.
2. This course not only cleanses, but also helps to lose weight.
3. The duration of the course is no more than 7 days.
4. A diet on fiber helps to eliminate the processes of fermentation and putrefaction in the digestive tract, normalizing cholesterol and blood sugar levels. Helps improve heart function, reduces the risk of gallstones.
5. The cleansing regimen is contraindicated in pregnancy, oncology, diseases of the gastrointestinal tract, mental disorders, and pregnancy.

# Make a menu based on following:

| Allowed foods | Limited (you can eat no more than 1-2 times a week) | Forbidden |
|---|---|---|
| legumes;<br>champignons;<br>baked goods made from wholemeal flour;<br>whole wheat bread;<br>buckwheat;<br>dried fruits;<br>millet;<br>flax seeds;<br>oats;<br>berries;<br>coarse wheat pasta;<br>fruits;<br>greenery;<br>nuts;<br>juices. | lean meat;<br>spices, seasonings;<br>honey;<br>steamed lean fish;<br>boiled eggs;<br>low-fat dairy products. | All products not listed in the permitted and restricted list. |

## Menu option

Example of a diet for two days:

| Meal | First day | Second day |
|---|---|---|
| Breakfast | 150 g of peach, pear and apple salad, 15 ml of natural yogurt, 2 tsp. flax seeds. | 200 g of oatmeal in water with dried fruits, 150 ml of green tea. |
| Lunch | 1 pear. | 1 grapefruit. |
| Lunch | 200 g of durum wheat pasta, 150 g of "Brush" salad. | 150 ml of squash soup, 100 g of boiled chicken breast. |
| Afternoon snack | 100 g of salad from grated raw carrots and beets. | 100 g of cabbage and cucumber salad. |
| Dinner | 200 g of brown rice and lentil pilaf, 150 g of vegetable salad with sprouted cereals. | 200 g buckwheat porridge, baked half an eggplant with garlic. |

# Diuretic diet

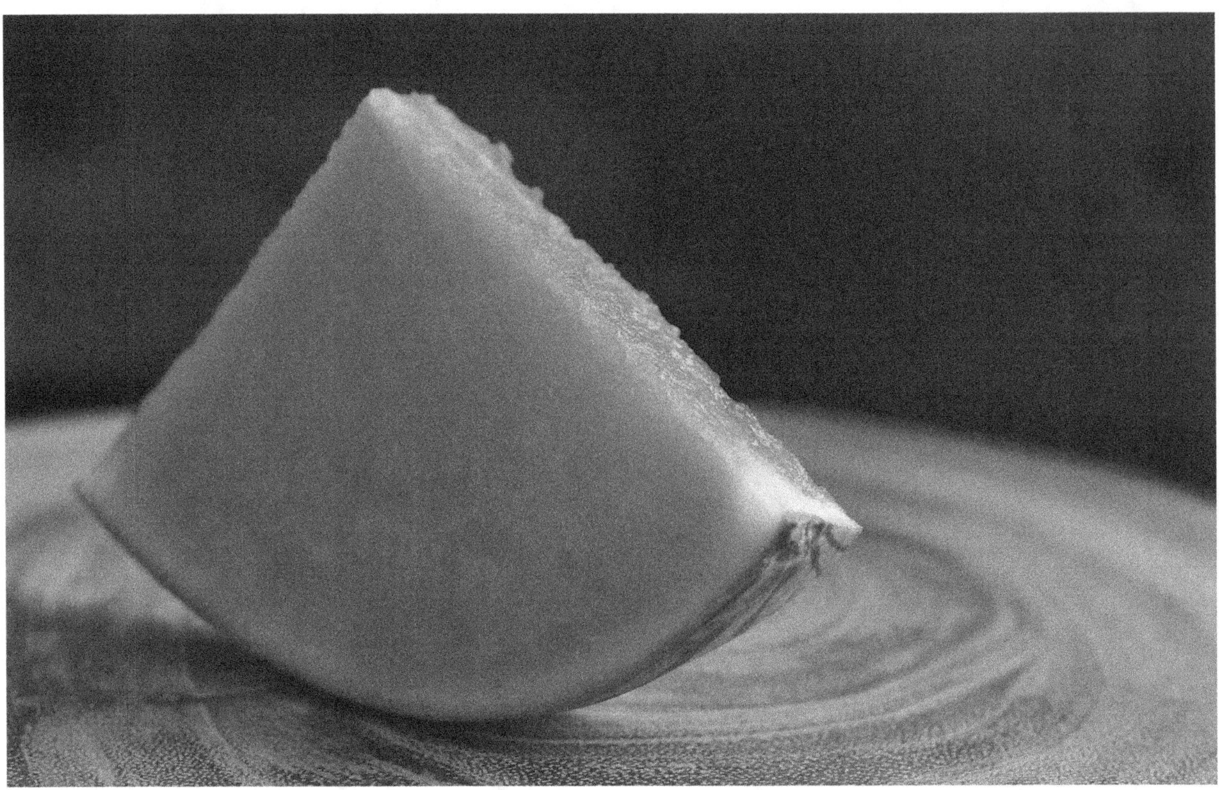

**The salt-free detox diet is the most popular among detoxifiere. Characteristics:**

1. It implies the use of diuretic products, vegetable and animal proteins. All food that retains fluid in the body is prohibited.
2. The cleansing regimen puts a lot of stress on the bladder and kidneys, so the menu must be composed correctly.
3. The diet is intended while sand in the kidneys, slagging of the body, swelling, excess weight.
4. The maximum duration is 3 days.
5. Contraindicated in renal failure.
6. Between meals, it is advisable to drink diuretic teas, freshly squeezed juices, and mineral water without gas. It is better to puree the dishes.

## Allowed and prohibited foods

The diet should be made using the following lists:

| Allowed foods | Limited (you can eat no more than 1-2 times a week) | Forbidden |
| --- | --- | --- |
| watermelon; | | |
| viburnum; | | |
| artichoke; | | |
| cranberry; | | |
| melon; | | |
| lingonberry; | | |
| green tea; | | |
| rosehip; | | |
| millet; | | bakery products; |
| gooseberry; | | eggs; |
| oats; | | yeast; |
| apple vinegar; | | crisps; |
| buckwheat; | legumes; | fried food; |
| spinach; | soy milk; | sauces; |
| ginger root; | Brown rice; | fatty fish; |
| pumpkin; | nuts; | salt; |
| onion; | shrimp; | smoked meats; |
| asparagus; | olive oil; | cream; |
| carrot; | squid; | red meat; |
| beet; | skim cheese; | wheat flour; |
| cucumbers; | oysters; | sweets; |
| black radish; | lean fish; | semi-finished products; |
| radish; | mussels; | mayonnaise; |
| any drinks except alcohol, soda | natural yogurt; | milk; |
| and energy drinks. | a hen. | margarine. |

**Example of a menu**

A variant of the diet for two days:

| Meal | First day | Second day |
| --- | --- | --- |
| **Breakfast** | 150 g of grated beets, 50 g of fresh berries. | 150 g grated carrots, a handful of walnuts. |
| **Lunch** | 200 g watermelon, 150 ml green tea with lemon and ginger. | 200 g melon, 150 ml freshly squeezed orange juice. |
| **Lunch** | 180 ml of carrot cream soup, 50 g of grated radish. | 180 ml of squash soup, 100 g of cucumber and radish salad. |
| **Afternoon snack** | 200 g of watermelon, 150 ml of oat kvass. | 200 g melon, 150 ml apple juice. |
| **Dinner** | 200 g buckwheat, 100 g tomato and bell pepper salad. | 200 g of rice, 100 g of cucumber and cabbage salad. |

# Diet for the intestines

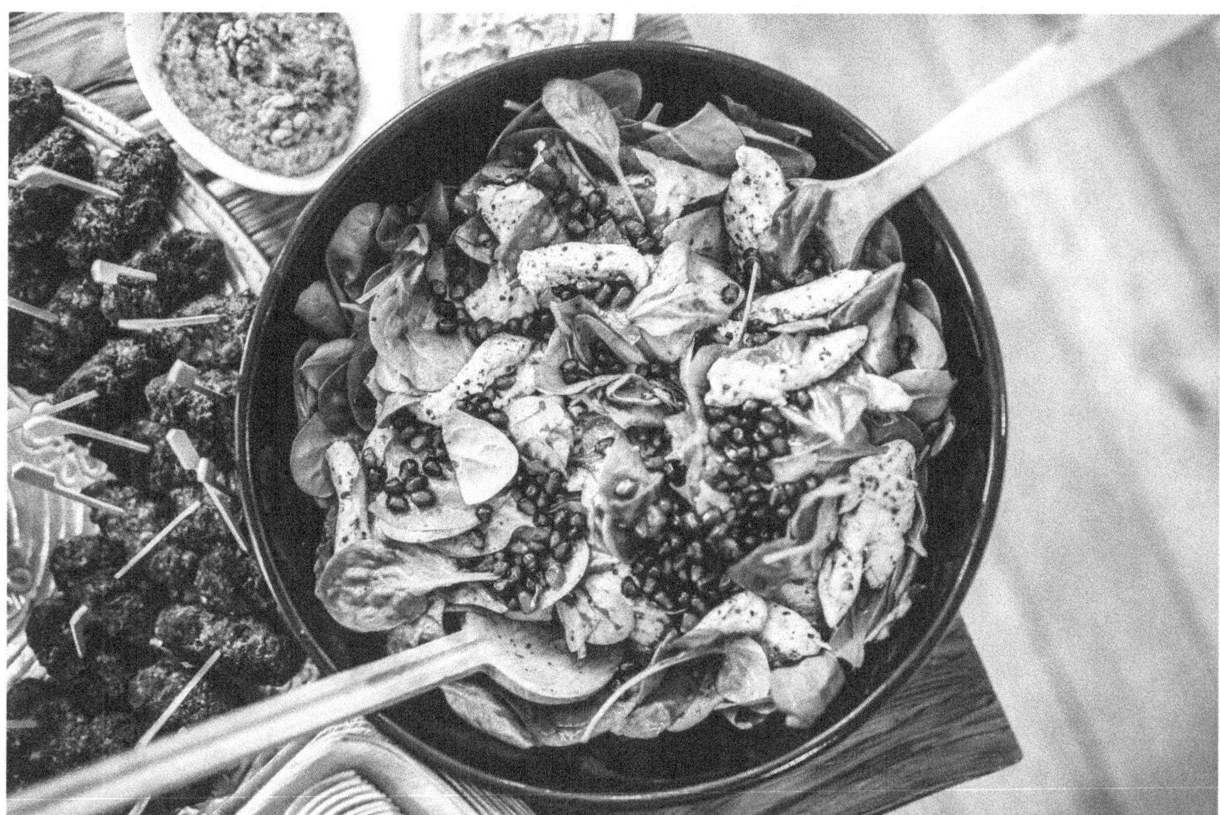

## Diet for cleansing the intestines

This food system helps to remove the accumulated feces, toxins. Features:

1. The basis of the diet are products that have a laxative effect. It liquefy feces, activate intestinal peristalsis. Products with an astringent and fixing effect are excluded.
2. The maximum duration is 3 days. Laxative products are addictive. If you use them constantly, dysbiosis will begin.
3. Contraindications - diseases of the gastrointestinal tract.

When planning a menu, be guided by the following lists:

| Allowed foods | Forbidden |
| --- | --- |
| <ul><li>spinach;</li><li>dairy products (especially sour milk, buttermilk, yogurt);</li><li>dried fruits;</li><li>seaweed;</li><li>beet juice;</li><li>oatmeal;</li><li>pumpkin;</li><li>cucumber pickle;</li><li>apricots;</li><li>vegetable oil;</li><li>beet;</li><li>plums;</li><li>carrot;</li><li>apples.</li></ul> | <ul><li>alcoholic drinks;</li><li>chocolate;</li><li>bananas;</li><li>spice;</li><li>pears;</li><li>fatty food;</li><li>barberry;</li><li>rich broth;</li><li>baking;</li><li>eggs;</li><li>rice porridge;</li><li>fatty fish;</li><li>semolina;</li><li>fat meat;</li><li>semi-finished products;</li><li>jelly;</li><li>spicy dishes;</li><li>canned food;</li><li>marinades;</li><li>smoked meats;</li><li>mayonnaise;</li><li>strong tea, coffee.</li></ul> |

**Sample menu**

**Diet option for two days:**

| Meal | First day | Second day |
|---|---|---|
| **Breakfast** | 200 g of oatmeal with prunes. | 200 g buckwheat, 50 g grated carrots. |
| **Lunch** | 5-6 pcs. prunes, 200 ml of beet-carrot juice (mix in equal proportions). | 1 apple, 200 ml of cucumber pickle. |
| **2 Lunch** | 180 ml of spinach cream soup, 100 g of grated beetroot salad with herbs and garlic. | 180 ml pumpkin puree soup, 100 g grated carrots. |
| **Afternoon snack** | 5-6 pcs. prunes, 200 ml of beet-carrot juice (mix in equal proportions). | 1 apple, 200 ml of cucumber pickle. |
| **Dinner** | 150 g of seaweed. | 150 g fat-free cottage cheese. |

# Porridge diet

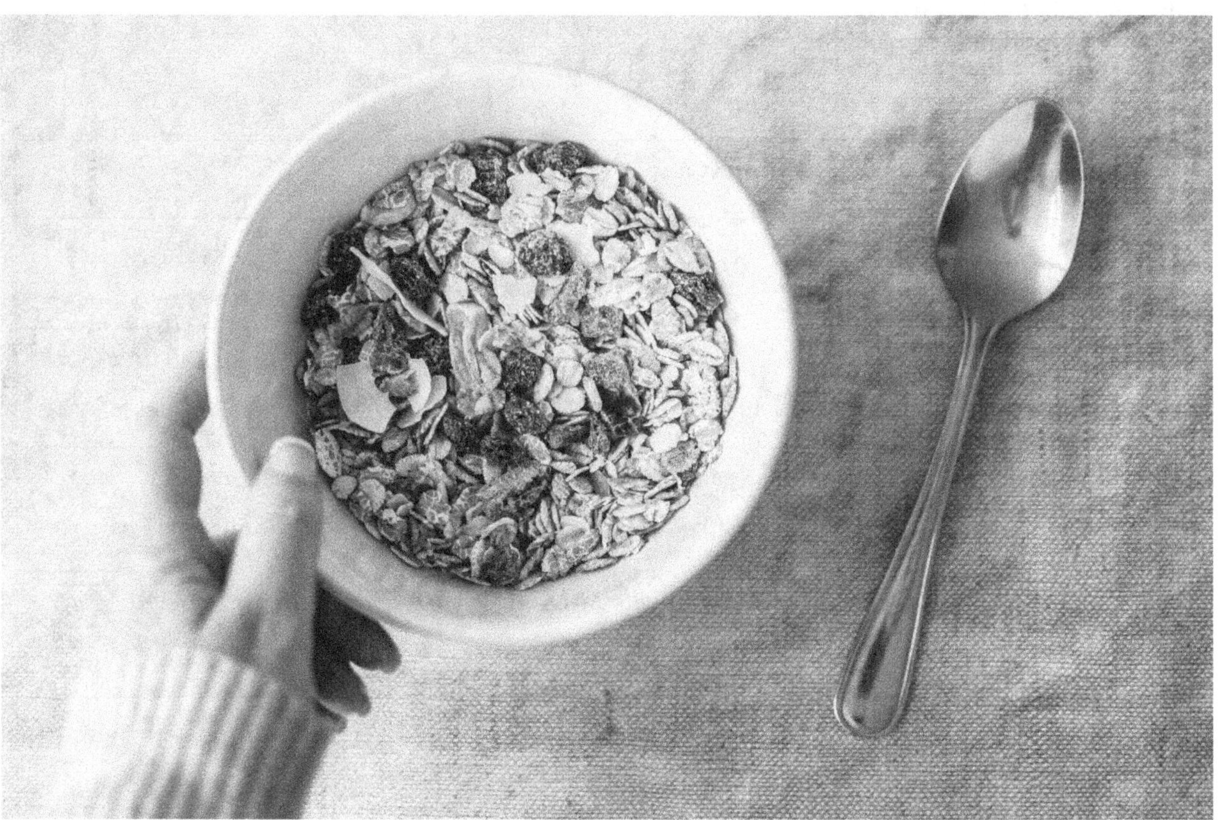

Dishes made from cereals help to remove toxins from the body. There are many diets on porridge.The basic principles are the same as other cleansing agents: consult a doctor, prepare the body, eat fractionally, observe a drinking regimen. Average duration is 3 to 14 days. The main types of diets on cereals for removing toxins:

- buckwheat;
- rice;
- oatmeal.

**Buckwheat**

It has a cleansing effect and helps to lose weight. Buckwheat saturates for a long time and contains a lot of vegetable protein. Features of the diet:

1. There are different options for the cleansing regime with a duration of 3 to 14 days.

2. Salt, sugar and products containing them, seasonings, sauces, spices must be completely excluded from the diet.

3. Allowed dietary salads from vegetables and herbs, all fruits except grapes and

bananas, eggs, low-calorie natural yogurts.

4.  It is strictly forbidden to eat after six in the evening.

The basis of the diet is buckwheat porridge. It is cooked like this:

1.  pour 100 g of cereal with 200 ml of boiling water.
2.  Wrap the container with a warm towel. Insist all night.
3.  You get about 250 g of steamed cereals.

There are three types of buckwheat diet:

1.  Strict. Only buckwheat is allowed for breakfast, lunch and dinner. The amount of porridge is any. Last meal 4 hours before bedtime. Duration - 3 days.
2.  buttermilk-buckwheat. You can eat any amount of cereals per day. You can drink 1 liter of buttermilk and water unlimited. Duration - 5 days.
3.  Lightweight. Duration - 2 weeks. Buckwheat, vegetables, fruits, dairy products, protein products of animal origin (lean fish, eggs, chicken and turkey breast, lean beef) are allowed.


**Rice**

This cleansing diet for weight loss is similar to buckwheat, but the total calories are lower. There is no gluten in rice. It is rich in potassium, B vitamins, lecithin, amino acids. Features of the cleansing regime:

1.  Duration - 1 week.
2.  Salt, sugar, spices, seasonings, flour, coffee, alcohol, potatoes, fatty, fried foods are prohibited.
3.  Allowed seafood, vegetables, fresh and dried fruits, green tea, still mineral water.
4.  All fatty, fried, salty foods, sweets and semi-finished products are prohibited.
5.  Raw and boiled vegetables and fruits are allowed.
6.  Contraindications: pregnancy, cardiovascular diseases, lactation, renal failure, colds, pathologies of the gastrointestinal tract.

The basis of the diet is properly cooked rice porridge. Recipe:

1. Rinse the rice. Soak overnight.
2. In the morning, pour cold water in a ratio of 1: 1.5.
3. Boil. Minimize the fire. Cook, covered, for 20 minutes.
4. Turn off. Let it brew for 10 minutes.

## Oatmeal

Oatmeal is rich with vitamins and minerals and contains few calories. Features of the diet:

1. Duration - 7 days.
2. Before starting a diet, it is recommended the procedure for cleansing the body with rice jelly.
3. Only oatmeal, low-fat dairy products, fruits are allowed.
4. Contraindications: damage to the skeletal system, pregnancy, celiac disease, lactation, allergy tendencies, renal failure, heart disease.
5. Do not drink the water, tea, coffee while eating oatmeal. Drinks are allowed half an hour after eating.

The basis of the diet is oatmeal. It is prepared without sugar, salt, oil. You can add honey, fruits, berries, ginger root, pepper, cinnamon. Recipe:

1. Pour cold water over oatmeal. The proportion is 1: 3.
2. Cook until a viscous consistency (about 15 minutes), or steam in a thermos for 3 hours.

# Mono-diets

## The Rice diet

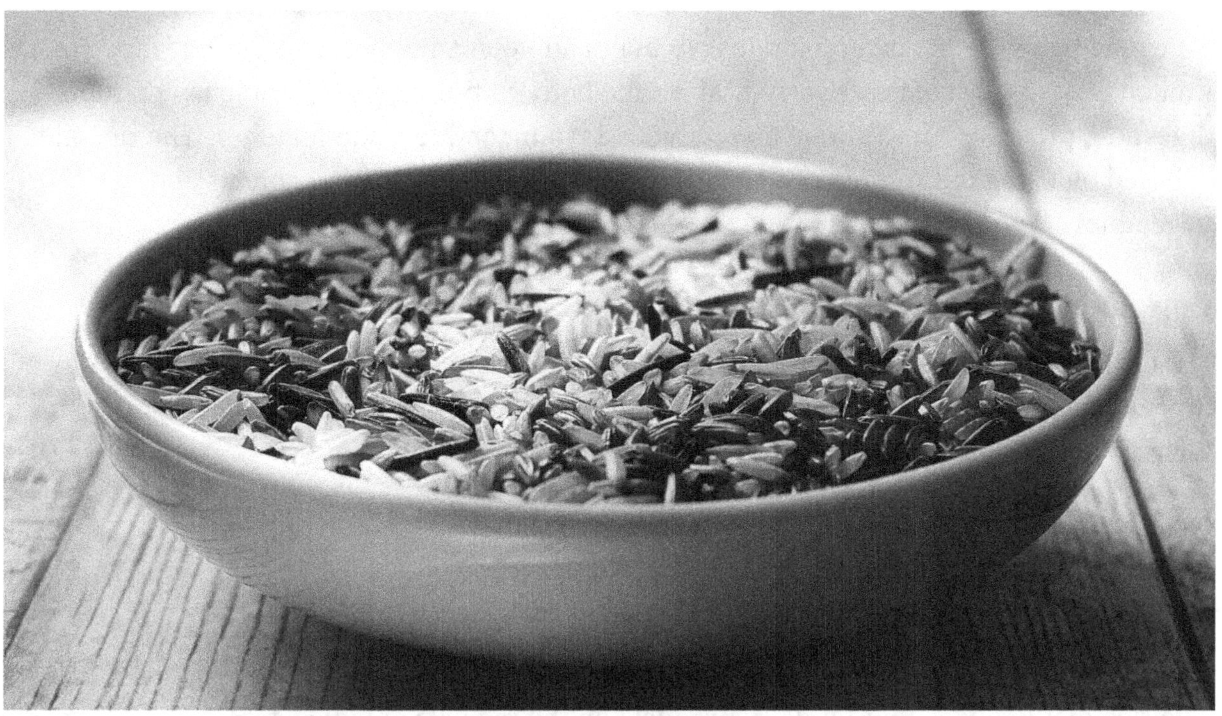

### Rice diet for weight loss and detoxification by day

Rice-based diet was developed by American doctors to treat heart and kidney diseases. The technique is effective in combating hypertension and obesity. The rice diet in different versions (3, 7, 30 days) is widely used, it really helps to lose excess weight. The hard way to lose weight has contraindications - before switching this diet, you need to consult a doctor.

### The essence of the diet

The basis of weight loss techniques is the use of carbohydrates and fiber which are found in rice grains, vegetables and fruits. The diet restricts using fat and salt. It is also necessary to monitor the calorie content of food. Recommendations for the daily diet:

- amount of salt - up to 1 g, fat - 22 g, protein - 20 g.
- caloric content of food - 800-1500 calories.

The rice diet can last from three days to a month. To be effective, those who are losing weight are advised to drink water and perform simple physical exercises. It is important to keep track of your onionel movements because rice can cause constipation.

To get energy, the body burns fat reserves during the diet. Rice has a low calorie content, quickly saturates, removes excess fluid and toxins, accelerates metabolism. The grains contain B vitamins, trace elements, 80% complex carbohydrates. Rice lacks the plant protein gluten, which causes allergies and intolerances in 1% of people.

## Lots of carbohydrates

Someone believes that carbohydrates are evil, and you can only lose weight if they are limited. These substances are essential for the body to function. Its deficiency disrupts digestion, processes in the brain and nervous system, and leads to lethargy. The rice diet is based on using the complex of carbohydrates, which are found in cereals and vegetables.

## Low fat and sodium

For normal functioning of the body, 0.5 g of salt containing sodium is required per day. Since this product retains fluid in the tissues and increases appetite, in order to lose weight, its use must be reduced. Salt restriction:

- normalizes blood pressure;
- improves kidney function;
- reduces weight by eliminating edema, fluid withdrawal.

The rice diet includes low-fat dairy products on the menu. Some vegetable oil is allowed. Banned:

- oily fish;
- pork;
- duck;
- offal.

## Diet principles

For effective weight loss on the rice technique, you need to follow the rules:

- First, spend a fasting day. Soak a glass of rice in the evening, boil it in the morning for 15 minutes and eat it in 6 meals. So you will evaluate the effect of the diet on your well-being, and you will get the first result - weight loss.
- Use only approved products, exclude anything that is prohibited.
- Start with a low daily calorie intake, gradually increase it taking into account the weight loss phase.
- Drink at least two liters of water a day to prevent constipation.
- The diet is prohibited for constipation, metabolic disorders, during pregnancy and

lactation.

- Before trying the technique, consult with your doctor, take basic tests. Make sure you are healthy.

## Allowed Foods

The rice porridge diet allows the use of fresh vegetables and fruits. Change it every day. During weight loss, the following types of products are:

- Lean fish, lean meat - chicken, beef.
- Whole grains and legumes.
- Low fat dairy products - buttermilk, yogurt, cottage cheese.
- Sunflower and olive oil.
- Freshly squeezed juices and green tea.

## White and brown rice

In this weight loss technique, it is important to choose the right staple. Often those who are losing weight for the duration of the diet choose white polished rice with a more pleasant taste. It cooks quickly, is available in all stores, and is affordable. Long grain varieties are believed to be healthier than round or chopped grains.

Brown rice has a shell that contains fiber and many useful substances. Such grains have a shorter shelf life and require prolonged heat treatment. After boiling, it remains harsher than white varieties.

## Forbidden foods

During the rice diet, do not eat canned food and convenience foods. Banned:

- Fatty meat and fish, sausages.
- Bread, any pastries and pastries.
- Condiments, sauces, hot spices, mayonnaise, marinades.
- Nuts and sweets, sugar, bananas, grapes.
- Alcohol, carbonated drinks, black tea and coffee.

**Weight loss phases**

The rice diet, if it is designed for three weeks, includes 3 stages:

- The first phase is detoxification. The basis is calorie restriction and the complete absence of salt.
- The second is the weight loss phase. The daily calorie content has been increased due to new products.
- The phase of consolidating the results. Weight loss is slowed down, it is important to maintain the effect obtained.

**Detoxification**

In the first phase of the rice diet, the greatest weight loss occurs. The daily calorie content is 800 calories. At this time, salt is completely forbidden, from cereals you can only eat rice and quinoa. Vegetables are allowed 6 times a week and fruits are allowed 1 day. Don't forget to drink water.

In this phase, the body actively removes fluid, salts and toxins, edema disappears, and blood pressure decreases. You may feel faint - this is a sign of successful detoxification. Monitor your condition: if you are not strong, it is better to rest, and if you have - add light exercise.

**Weight Loss**

The second phase of the rice diet is the vegetarian eating period. It lasts a week, if you feel well, you can extend it for one more. Calorie content increased to 1000 calories.

> *The diet includes legumes, low-fat dairy products, which should be eaten 5 times a week.*

Lean fish allowed on weekends. Eat vegetables raw.

**Consolidation of results**

The last stage - the phase of weight maintenance - lasts 7 days. Daily calorie intake has been increased to 1500 calories by adding meat and fish Deuce a week. To consolidate the result, continue to eat vegetables, if you want, fill them with vegetable oil. Include cottage cheese, nuts, cheese in the diet.

After finishing the rice diet, it is important to smoothly move on to your usual diet. The transition period lasts 7-10 days. Gradually increase the calorie content of your food. Add broths, salt, cereals. To stabilize your weight, take a fasting day on rice once a week.

**The effectiveness of the diet**

You can lose about 10 kilograms in a month using a rice diet.

*The body is cleansed of toxins, the work of organs improves - mainly the kidneys and heart.*

Losing weight passes away bouts of hypertension, lower cholesterol and blood sugar levels. Nutritionists recommend this as a short term weight loss method.

**Advantages and Disadvantages**

Positive aspects of a rice diet:

- A large amount of fiber in vegetables creates a feeling of fullness, normalizes onionel function.
- Excess fluid leaves the body, toxins are removed.
- The edema disappears, the pressure stabilizes, the pain in the joints decreases.
- Vitamins and microelements in rice improve heart function.
- In a short period, you lose significant body weight.

The disadvantages of the diet include low calorie content, which causes weakness, decreased performance. Not everyone can tolerate severe nutritional restrictions. Cons of the rice diet:

- The presence of contraindications.
- Loss of muscle mass - protein foods are scarce.
- With long-term use, it removes useful microelements and vitamins from the body. Take drugs or supplements with these substances.
- Difficulty following the methodology on weekdays, outside the home.
- Long-term diet requires a careful approach, medical supervision.

**Sample Menu**

A good option is a three-day rice diet. It is not so difficult, but it also helps to get rid of extra pounds. An approximate weight loss menu is pre-scheduled for all meals.

**First day:**

- Breakfast. Rice porridge (portion - 70 g), a glass of yogurt, an apple.
- Lunch. Cucumber, tomato, cabbage salad, seasoned with olive oil - 120 g. Boiled rice - 150 g, green tea.
- Dinner. Grilled zucchini - 100 g, rice - 150 g, buttermilk - 250 ml.

**Second day:**

- Breakfast. Rice with lemon juice - 100 g, orange, green tea.
- Lunch. Fresh carrot salad - 120 g, boiled rice - 150 g, pear.
- Dinner. Cabbage stewed with onions and herbs - 100 g, rice porridge - 150 g, a glass of yogurt without additives.

**Third day:**

- Breakfast. Rice with raisins - 50 g, cottage cheese seasoned with sour cream - 50 g, green tea.
- Lunch. Vegetable pilaf - 270 g, apple, glass of milk.
- Dinner. Rice stewed with zucchini and tomatoes - 250 g, buttermilk - 250 ml.

# The Potato diet

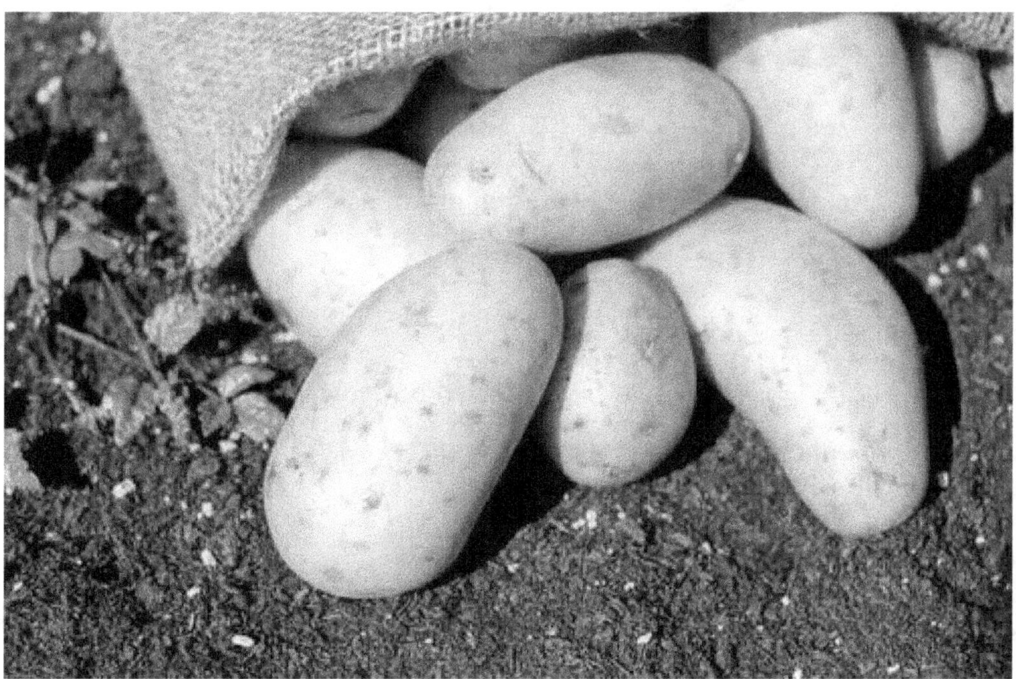

## Potato diet for weight loss: menu with recipes

Weight loss method is ideal for people who are not ready for tough dietary restrictions. Dieting, you will practically not feel hungry. The exception is a strict 3-day program on one potato or with vegetables, buttermilk. Following the recommendations, you can lose from 0.5 to 2 kg of excess weight daily.

## The essence of the potato diet

For effective weight loss, adhere to the basic rules:

1. Use boiled, baked or steamed potatoes in their skins.
2. Eat fractionally small meals.
3. Observe the regime. Eat at regular intervals. Have dinner 2-3 hours before bedtime.
4. Drink 2–3 liters of clean water daily.
5. Eliminate salt or use it in a minimal amount - up to 2-3 g per day.

## Is it possible to lose weight on potatoes

The benefits of a potato are explained by its rich composition.

It contains:

- minerals - phosphorus, sodium, magnesium, iodine, iron, cobalt, copper, calcium;
- vitamins - especially A, C, group B;
- vegetable protein;
- cellulose.

For weight loss, such characteristics of potatoes are important as:

- age (young or old);
- the presence of heat treatment (raw or cooked);
- cooking method (boiled, baked, fried, fried; peeled or peeled; without or with additives; whole or chopped).

Depending on the processing method, the calorie content of the product changes. 100 ml of potato juice and 100 g of raw vegetable contains 76 kcal, boiled "little brown" - 82 kcal, baked in a peel - 85–92 kcal; in the form of puree on water - 90 kcal.

*When losing weight, exclude fried potatoes, chips, mashed potatoes with butter, milk, dressings in the form of fatty sauces from the diet.*

Potatoes are a high glycemic food (70 units and up), but some cooking methods reduce their GI. If you are overweight, it is better to eat it raw (Japanese salads), steam it, boil it or bake it in a peel. Cooking tubers completely reduces the glycemic index by 10-15 units.

Losing weight will be effective when using small to medium-sized young potatoes with a minimum of fat, "fast" carbohydrates, solanine. Early root vegetables have less starch, but a lot of vegetable protein, so you can get enough of the tubers.

*On a strict potato diet, you can lose 1–2 kg of excess weight a day. On a gentle program, about 0.5 kg per day is consumed.*

Why is it valuable to use potatoes when dieting:

- excess fluid is removed;
- the nervous system is strengthened, brain function improves;
- due to the presence of potassium, the work of the cardiovascular system is

normalized;

- digestion improves, intestinal functionality is improved (if you cook a vegetable in a peel and eat it cold);
- vitamin C improves tissue regeneration, so it helps to quickly restore muscles after intense workouts;
- due to the presence of ascorbic acid, immunity is strengthened.

## Advantages and disadvantages of the potato diet

The main advantages of the weight loss program:

- delicious and easy-to-prepare meals;
- there is no hunger, lethargy, decreased performance;
- the budget is saved - the root crop is inexpensive.

## Disadvantages of a hearty potato diet for weight loss:

- blood sugar increases, so the technique is not suitable for diabetics;
- a poor diet requires additional intake of vitamin complexes;
- provokes constant thirst, therefore, before and after meals, you need to drink a glass of still water.

## Potato Diet Options

There are short-term, strict programs and more gentle systems designed for 1–2 weeks. Fasting day on potatoes or 3-5-day diet options help to get rid of 1-5 extra pounds. Programs are relevant if you urgently need to lose weight by a certain date. Potato diets for 1–2 weeks are suitable for gradual weight loss without much stress on the body. Recommended for overweight people over 10 kg.

## A strict three-day diet

It takes 1-2 kg per day. Features of the potato mono diet:

- Eat 1 kg of potato tubers per day. There should be 6 meals. Serving size is about 150 g.
- Use baked or boiled potatoes without oil, salt and spices. Add fresh herbs for flavor.
- Drink clean water, tea, chicory.

**Potato-buttermilk diet**

Duration - 3-5 days. It takes 2-5 kg of excess weight. The result depends on the initial parameters of the figure, the metabolic rate and the strictness of adherence to the dietary rules. Features of nutrition:

- Use low-fat buttermilk. Replace it with homemade low-calorie yogurt (up to 1.5%) if necessary.
- Supplement the menu with baked or boiled potatoes without oil, spices, vegetable salads.
- You can use potato juice for weight loss. To do this, grate the tubers on a fine grater, squeeze the liquid through cheesecloth, leave for 10-15 minutes. Drink without starchy residue.
- Repeat the potato diet after 1.5–2 months if necessary.

**Approximate 3-day menu:**

- Day 1. Breakfast - 1 tbsp. buttermilk. Lunch - 4 medium boiled potatoes. Dinner - 1 tbsp. buttermilk, 1 baked potato.
- Day 2. Breakfast - 1 tbsp. buttermilk. Lunch - baked potatoes (200 g). Dinner - carrot and cabbage salad with lemon juice (150 g), 1 tbsp. buttermilk.
- Day 3. Breakfast - 2 tbsp. yoghurt. Lunch - potato casserole (150 g), cucumber and greens salad (150 g). Dinner - 1 tbsp. buttermilk, boiled potatoes (150 g).

**Two-week meal plan for effective weight loss**

In 14 days on a potato diet, you will get rid of 7-9 kg.

Nutrition nuances:

- About 1 kg of potatoes per day, dividing it into 6 meals. Serving size is about 150 g.
- Drink clean water from liquids.
- For the first 3 days, eat baked potatoes without salt, spices and oil.
- For the next week, eat boiled or baked potatoes with salt and olive oil.
- For the next 4 days, reduce the serving size to 100 g. Mix mashed potatoes with oil, salt, herbs, spices or lemon juice.

**Rapid weight loss on a potato and cabbage diet**

The duration of the weight loss program is a week. Leaves up to 7 kg of excess weight. Features of weight loss:

- Eat 4-5 medium-sized potatoes per day. They can be boiled or baked.
- Eat 500 g of cabbage per day - fresh, stewed or steamed.
- Drink unsweetened teas and still mineral water from liquids.
- Don't use salt or spices other than pepper and garlic.

**Potato diet dishes**

Soups, mashed potatoes, baked, boiled vegetables with lemon juice, herbs - not all options for wholesome food. Add simple, low-calorie potato dishes to your diet.

**Potatoes with tomato sauce**
1. Boil 5 medium potatoes with peel.
2. Chop and mix 2 tomatoes, 2-3 cloves of garlic, a bit of fresh herbs.
3. Slice potatoes into rings, combine with tomato dressing.
4. Add black pepper if necessary.

**Baked potatoes with herbs, garlic**
1. Peel, chop 0.5 kg of potatoes.
2. Grate 2-3 cloves of garlic, mix with vegetables.
3. Transfer to a baking dish. Put in an oven preheated to 200 degrees for half an hour.
4. Decorate the finished dish with fresh herbs.

**Stewed potatoes**
1. Peel and wash 1 kg potatoes, 1 carrot.
2. Cut vegetables into circles, place in a saucepan, cover with water. Place on medium heat.
3. After 20 minutes, add the tomato sliced into circles. Simmer for another 10 minutes.
4. Sprinkle the finished dish with chopped herbs.

**Diet is not suitable for:**

pregnant women, lactating mothers, children and the elderly with obesity. If you are a lot overweight, be sure to consult with your doctor. Potatoes for weight loss are contraindicated in the following conditions:

- gastrointestinal disorders - heartburn, flatulence, bloating, belching, nausea, vomiting, diarrhea and constipation;
- urolithiasis;
- diabetes mellitus;
- liver disease;
- hypotension;
- low acidity of the stomach;
- individual intolerance.

# The Orange diet

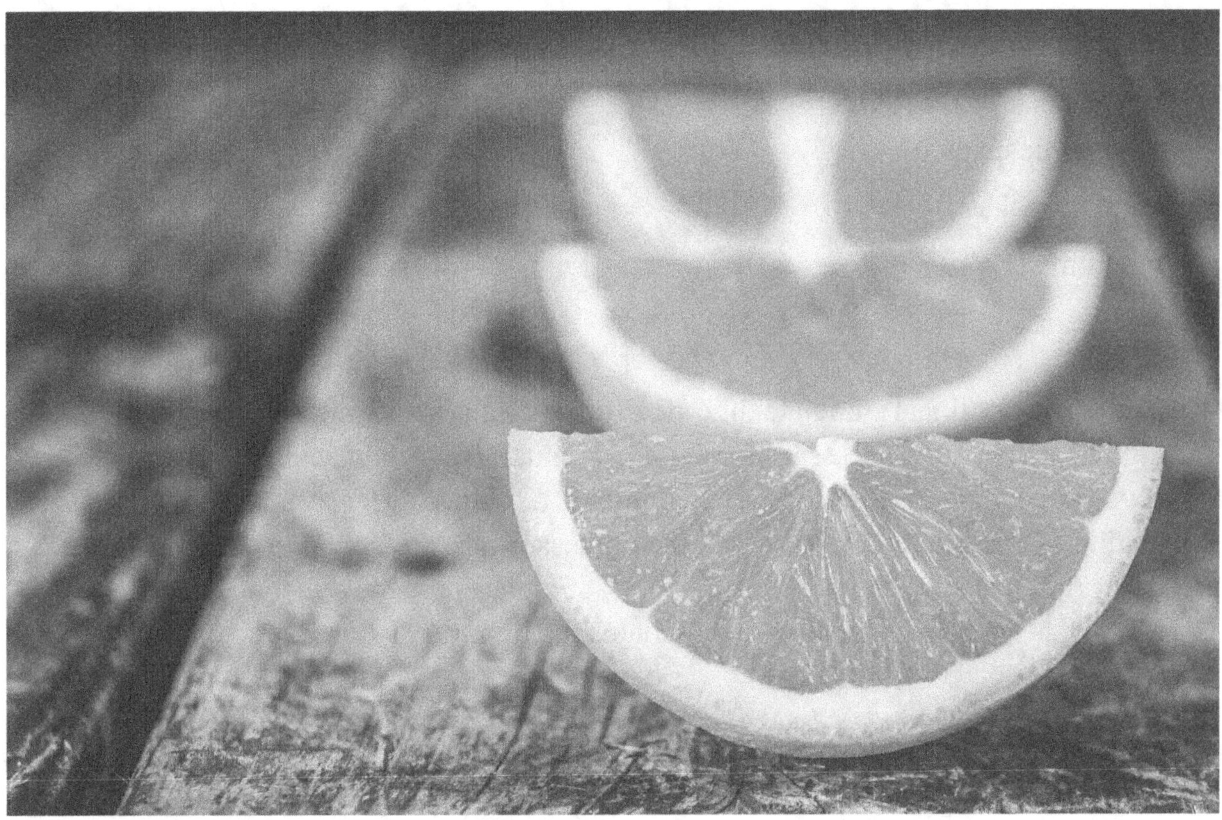

## Orange diet: menu options

Any citruses have powerful antioxidant and anti-stress properties, rich with vitamin C and fiber. The low calorie content of oranges allows you to use it for weight loss and health improvement. An orange diet can help you to lose extra pounds without feeling hungry or exercising.

## Is it possible to lose weight on oranges?

Citrus has  low calorie content (35 kcal / 100 g),  and lack of fat. Carbohydrates from the orange (there is still more fiber) are not processed into lipids, so someone who has eaten an orange does not want to eat for about 2–4 hours. Orange is extremely useful for snacks, weight loss. Due to the essential oils in the peel and pulp, mood improves, and vitality increases.

## The chemical composition and beneficial properties of the orange:

In oranges - less than 1% of proteins, only 8.1% of carbohydrates. The glycemic index of the product (GI) is 45 units (it can vary between varieties).

It contain:

- vitamins of group B, A, C, PP;
- calcium, phosphorus, iron, sodium, magnesium;
- sugar;
- organic acids;
- phytoncides;
- aroma oils;
- pectins.

The fruit's dietary fibers stimulate digestion. Fiber cleanses the intestines, gives the feeling of satiety that is necessary for losing weight. Due to folic acid in citruses, oranges improve skin condition. Freshly squeezed juice will reduce the secretion of bile, preventing constipation. Due to pectin, the processes of putrefaction in the intestines are stopped - the substance envelops the contents, stimulates the movement of the masses. Organic acids are also beneficial - it stimulates the burning of stored fat.

## Types of diets with oranges

Nutritionists distinguish several options for losing weight on citrus fruits.

| Type | Features, effectiveness | Duration, days |
|---|---|---|
| Egg-orange diet | For breakfast - boiled eggs and orange juice. There are 3 doses per day.<br>You can lose weight by 2-3 kg. | 5 |
| Orange and chicken | For breakfast - boiled eggs and orange juice, for lunch - fillet of meat, for dinner - orange.<br>You will be able to lose 5-7 kg. | 14 |
| On smoothies and orange juice | Fasting day - they drink orange juice, a lot of water, it is allowed to make smoothies with grapefruit.<br>Weight loss by 1-2 kg. | 1 |
| Buttermilk-orange | Buttermilk for breakfast, lunch and dinner, orange - for breakfast and dinner. Useful chicken breast, which can be baked, bread.<br>It will turn out to lose 3-4 kg. | 5 |

**Orange Diet for weight loss.**

| Pros | Cons |
| --- | --- |
| Vitamin C helps to cleanse the body of harmful substances and toxins, fight radicals, prevent aging | Heartburn may develop, gastritis may begin |
| Useful fiber helps not to feel hunger longer | Imbalanced diet, little proteins |
| Metabolism Activated | Too difficult to follow a varied diet |
| Rapid loss weight The | lost kilograms will return faster. |

**Principles of nutrition with an orange diet:**

- citruses are eaten fresh with pulp;
- freshly squeezed juice is diluted in half with water;
- in the heat, it is useful to make a refreshing lemonade from orange slices with ice;
- oranges are eaten after the main meal;
- It is not recommended to eat fruits late in the evening, they can slow down weight loss. Better to replace them with 100 ml of juice before dinner.

**Menu for 3 days**

With this diet, you can lose 2-3 kg. In addition to oranges, bread, tea, coffee, buttermilk, yogurt, fresh tomatoes, lean meat (beef, chicken fillet) are allowed.

**Sample menu:**

| Day | Breakfast | Lunch | Dinner |
|---|---|---|---|
| 1 | orange, a cup of tea | A bunch of greens, a tomato, bread, 250 ml of buttermilk | Tomato, a glass of yogurt, an orange |
| 2 | | Greens, an egg, a tomato, a loaf of bread, 250 ml of buttermilk | Tomato, 250 ml of yogurt, an orange, an egg |
| 3 | | Greens, 100 g of beef, tomato, bread, a glass of buttermilk | 100 g of beef, tomato, 250 ml of yogurt, orange, egg |
| 4 | | | |
| 5 | 400 g of cottage cheese for the whole day, water, green tea | | |
| 6 | | | |
| 7 | Boiled or steamed fish - 150 g, three times in day | | |

## Orange diet for 4 weeks

For a month of compliance with this diet, you can lose weight by 10 kg. The menu can be repeated by week: the

- first week - 1 kg of oranges, 2 boiled eggs, 2 liters of water daily;
- the second - 1 kg of citrus fruits, buckwheat in water without oil and salt, 2 liters of water daily;
- the third - 1 kg of oranges, fresh vegetables, fruits;
- the fourth - 1 kg of fruit, eggs, lean meat.

Starting from the third week, the entire proposed diet is divided into three equal doses, during the breaks they drink a lot of water and green tea without sugar. For breakfast, an orange and 2 boiled eggs. Sample menu for 24 days:

| Day | Lunch | Dinner |
|---|---|---|
| 1 | 200 g of fruit, except for banana, orange | 200 g of boiled meat |
| 2 | 200 g of boiled chicken | 200 g of vegetable salad (except for beets, carrots, potatoes), croutons, orange |
| 3 | Toast, 2 tomatoes, 150 g low-fat cheese | 200 g boiled beef |
| 4 | 200 g fruit | |
| 5 | 2 eggs, 200 g baked vegetables | |
| 6 | 200 g fruit | 200 g meat and 100 g grilled vegetables |
| 7 | 100 g chicken, 100 g vegetables, tomato, orange | 200 g vegetables, orange |
| 8 | 200 g of meat | 2 eggs, salad, orange |
| 9 | | |
| 10 | 100 g of chicken, 150 g of cucumbers | 2 eggs, orange |
| 11 | 2 eggs, 70 g of low-fat cheese, 100 g of boiled vegetables | |
| 12 | 200 g of steamed fish | 2 eggs |
| 13 | 200 g of boiled meat, orange | 200 g fruit salad |
| 14 | 50 g cucumbers and tomatoes each, 1 100 g boiled vegetables, 100 g boiled chicken, orange | Fruit salad (except for bananas, grapes, dates) - 200 g |
| 15 | Fruits until full, except for banana, mango, figs, grapes | |
| 16 | Boiled, steamed or fresh vegetables until satiety, excluding potatoes | |
| 17 | Fruits and vegetables from previous days | |
| 18 | Boiled fish (100 g per reception), 200 g of white cabbage salad at a time | |
| 19 | 175 g of steamed meat (chicken, beef, rabbit), 200 g of vegetable salad | |
| 20 | Fruits until you feel full | |

| 21 | |
|----|---|
| 22 | 3 tomatoes, 4 cucumbers , ¼ part of skinless chicken, can of canned tuna in oil, toast, orange |
| 23 | 4 cucumbers, 3 tomatoes, 200 g chicken, toast, orange |
| 24 | 2 cucumbers, 2 tomatoes, 1 tbsp. l. cottage cheese, 400 g boiled vegetables, bread, orange |
| 25 | Half chicken without skin (steamed), 1 cucumber, 3 tomatoes, orange, toast |
| 26 | 3 tomatoes, 2 soft-boiled eggs, 200 g of vegetable salad, orange - eat in equal portions |
| 27 | 400 grilled chicken fillet, 125 g cottage cheese, orange, 2 cucumbers and tomatoes, a glass of yogurt, toast |
| 28 | 2 cucumbers, 2 tomatoes, 400 g boiled vegetables, 30 g cottage cheese, toast, 200 g boiled fish |

## How to get out of the diet

Correct completion of the restrictive period will reduce the stress of losing weight. The end is made in stages:

- within two days after observing the restrictions, eat vegetable decoctions;

- after 4 days, soups, potatoes, cereals are introduced;

- a week later, non-dietary meats, starchy vegetables, sweet fruits, and dairy products are introduced.

## Contraindications

The orange diet is not for everyone. The most frequent contraindications to its observance:

- peptic ulcer diseases of the digestive system - even diluted sour juice can aggravate the condition, provoking exacerbations;

- allergy to any citrus fruits - to avoid complications;

- diabetes mellitus - sugar in fruits increases glucose levels;

- diseases of the cardiovascular system - with them, any severe restriction of nutrition threatens to deteriorate;

- pregnancy, lactation - the risk of abnormal development of the fetus or the occurrence of allergies in the baby;

- severe liver and kidney diseases - creating a high load on the organs threatens to worsen the condition.

# The Apple diet

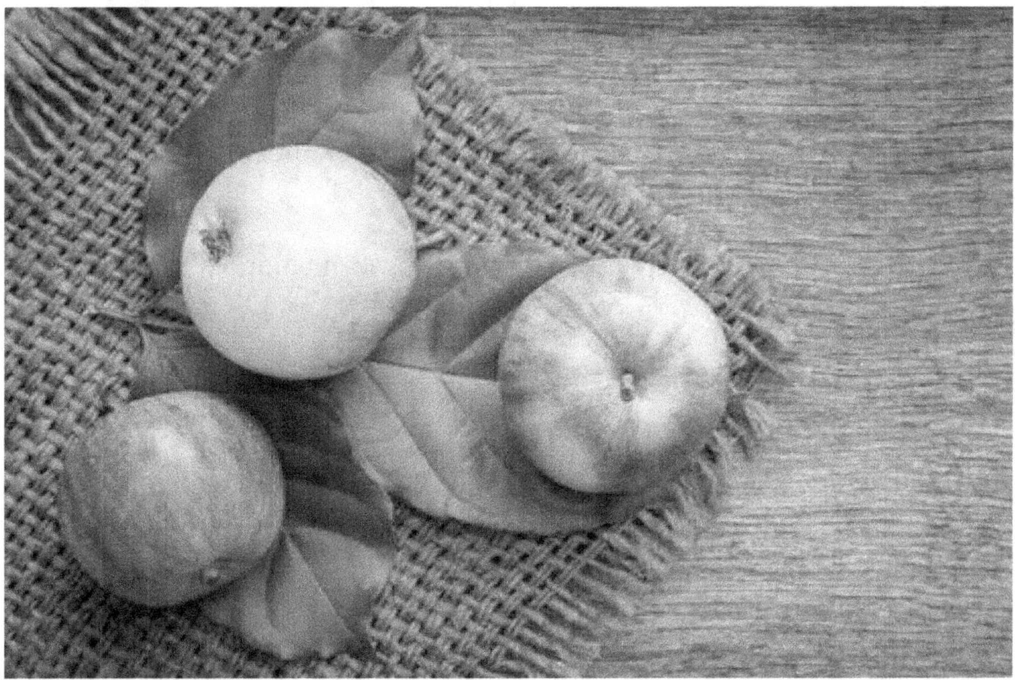

In the last century, it was considered that people gain weight due to the consumption of large amounts of animal fats, and the solution to the problem hides in the observance of fruit mono-diets. Later, the assumption was not confirmed, but weight loss on fruits alone remained very popular. Among them is an effective diet with an apple menu.

## The benefits of apples for the body

The diet on green apples is followed by many losing weight, and the reason for its popularity lies in its high efficiency and availability of fruits. It is suitable not only for healthy people, but also for those who have any diseases. Although there are still some contraindications. In addition to weight loss, the apple diet provides other benefits to the body, which are due to the presence of many valuable substances in fruits:

1. Pectin. It normalizes blood sugar, absorbs toxic, radioactive substances, metals, harmful acids, unnecessary fats, creates conditions favorable for the life of beneficial microorganisms.
2. Vitamin A. Improves eyesight, protects the body from colds.
3. Vitamin B2. Increases appetite, normalizes digestion processes, strengthens the nervous system.
4. Vitamin C. A large amount is found in sour varieties of fruits, relieves puffiness, prevents anemia, vitamin deficiency, and the penetration of infections into the

body.

5. Phosphorus. Fights insomnia, improves brain function.

6. Iodine. Eating just 5 apple seeds will provide you with a daily intake of iodine, which is necessary to prevent thyroid problems, improve brain activity.

7. Iron. A trace element, indispensable for the prevention and elimination of anemia, is very useful for children and pregnant women.

8. Organic acids. Eliminate bloating, flatulence, suppress fermentation processes in the intestines.

## Apple diet for weight loss

The weight loss apple-technique "promises" getting rid of 2-3 to 7-10 extra pounds, depending on its duration. This efficiency is due to the low calorie content of fruits, as well as an ability to remove excess water, toxins from the body, accelerate metabolic and digestive processes. The main thing is to strictly follow the rules of the diet, eat only permitted foods and exclude prohibited ones.

## Rules and principles

- Choose a suitable variety of fruit, preferably green and sour. Green apples contain few sugars and are not as allergenic as the sweet. In addition, acidic fruits contain more organic acids, dietary fiber that help break down fat. The following type of apples is considered the most suitable for a diet - it's a Granny Smith.

- Eat the fruit along with the skin, it contains a lot of fiber, which is indispensable for losing weight.

- Give preference to domestic apple varieties, imported ones are often processed with various substances to increase shelf life. It is easy to check the usefulness of the fruit when buying: swipe gently over its surface with your finger or nail. If the plaque disappears, do not take the product.

- Do not eat apples at night. Regardless of the variety, it contains a lot of fructose, which gives the body energy. During sleep, energy reserves are not consumed, but deposited in fats. If there is a strong sense of hunger, nutritionists recommend eating a little cottage cheese with a low percentage of fat.

- Don't forget to stay hydrated. The liquid will help cleanse the intestines and make the diet more effective.

- The way out of the apple weight loss system must be correct. It is still worth giving up junk food: sweet, smoked, salty, etc. The calorie intake should be increased gradually: by 25% in the first week, by 50% in the second, by 60-70% by the end of 3-4 weeks ...
- For best results, exercise during the apple menu diet.

## Do's and Don'ts of the Apple Diet

The most important thing you need during your diet is apples -  You need to eat an apple daily, raw or baked (depending on the type of fruit weight loss). In addition, it is important to adhere to the recommendations on how to diversify the diet, and what should be abandoned:

- If it is difficult to adhere strictly to the apple menu, there is always a feeling of hunger and feeling unwell, you can diversify the diet with cottage cheese, walnuts, eggs, vegetables (carrots, beets ), rice, green tea.
- It is imperative to exclude fatty, salty, fried foods, smoked meats, sweets, flour products, sauces, alcoholic and sweet carbonated drinks from the diet.

## How to lose weight on apples

There are several options for fruit weight loss: buttermilk-apple, medicinal, three-day apple mono-diet, fasting day on water and apples, diet for 7 days, etc. Each method of weight loss has its own duration and  effectiveness. Before you choose one of the diets with an apple menu, it is recommended to get tested and consult a doctor.

## Unloading day of apples and water

During fasting days, a hard cleansing of the body proceeds, the removal of excess fluid, toxins and blood thinning. Water fills your stomach, suppressing hunger, so you eat less and don't run out. The main thing is to drink water at room temperature, in small sips, at least 1.5 liters per day. An approximate apple menu for a diet with water can be as follows:

| Food intake | What to eat |
| --- | --- |
| 1/2 hour before breakfast, drink 0.35 liters of water, 1/3 hour before lunch - 0.3 liters, 1/3 hour before each snack and dinner - 0.2 liters each. | |
| **Breakfast** | <ul><li>apples (1–2 pcs.);</li><li>unsweetened tea;</li></ul> |
| **2 breakfast, lunch** | <ul><li>apple (1 pc.);</li></ul> |
| **Lunch** | <ul><li>apples (2-3 pcs., Can be baked);</li><li>unsweetened tea;</li></ul> |
| **Bakeddinner** | <ul><li>apple(1 pc.);</li><li>herbal tea.</li></ul> |

**For 3 days**

Doctors do not recommend following mono-methods of losing weight for more than 3-4 days in a row. The apple diet for 3 days just does not exceed the permissible period, therefore it will not harm health and the body. It is not easy to withstand the apple diet, but a plumb line of 3 kg is worth it. For better assimilation, fruits are allowed to grate. Also, don't forget about water balance. A three-day apple diet menu can be:

| Meals / day | 1 | 2 | 3 |
|---|---|---|---|
| **Breakfast** | Peeled fruits (2 pcs.) | | |
| **Lunch** | Grated fruits (2 pcs.) + Cinnamon (1 tsp.) | Peeled apples (2 pcs.) | Dried fruits (50 g) |
| **Dinner** | Purified apples (2 pcs.) | baked apple puree (2 pcs.) + cinnamon | baked apples (2 pcs.) + cinnamon |
| **before bedtime** | Purified apples (1 pc.) | | |

**For 7 days**

For best results of weight loss is recommended for a weak apple's diet. It's more satisfying and "promises" of 7-10 kg weight loss. The diet of this method is more varied, it contains rice, low-fat cottage cheese, vegetables, honey and nuts. In addition to the listed products, you need to drink 1.5–2 liters of pure water, herbal teas and green tea. A seven-day apple menu can be structured like this:

| Days / Meals | Breakfast | Lunch | Dinner |
| --- | --- | --- | --- |
| 1 | applesauce of 2-3 fruits; walnuts (2-3 pcs.); | puréed 2 carrots and 3 apples; | apple (3 pcs.); |
| 2 | apples (3 pcs.); boiled rice (0.1 kg); | fruits (bake in the oven) - 3 pcs.; | boiled rice (0.1 kg); apple (1 pc.); |
| 3 | fruits (2 pcs.); low-fat cottage cheese (0.1 kg); | apple (3 pcs.); cottage cheese (0%); nuts (2-3 pcs.); honey (1/2 tsp.); | low-fat cottage cheese (50 g); apple (1 pc.); |
| 4 | puree from 2 carrots and 1 fruit; | salad (2 apples + 1 carrots + 1 teaspoon honey); | baked fruits (3 pcs.); |
| 5 | apple (1 pc.); oatmeal (0.1 kg); | fruit and vegetable salad (1 boiled beet + 1 carrot + 1 apple); | 1 egg (hard boiled); fruits (2 pcs.); |
| 6 | fruits (3 pcs.); boiled rice (0.1 kg); | baked apples (3 pcs.); | apple (1 pc.); boiled rice (0.1 kg); |
| 7 | puree from 2 carrots and 1 apple. | apples (2 pcs.); carrots (1 pc.); honey (1 tsp). | baked fruits (3 pcs.). |

**Healing on baked apples**

The diet with baked apples is considered more gentle than other types of diets on fresh fruits. During it, there is a cleansing of toxins, the breakdown of fatty deposits and an improvement in metabolism.

The advantage of thermally processed fruits is that it's not irritate the walls of the stomach, which happens when fresh apples are consumed due to the content of fruit acids in them. You need to bake the fruit in its pure form, but if there is a strong hunger, you can put a filling made of berries or low-fat cottage cheese with honey. This dish is allowed only for breakfast or lunch.

Sticking to the apple menu with baked apples should be from 2-3 days to a maximum of a week, the plumb line in 2 days will be about 2 kg. There are three options for weight loss, which are recommended to alternate: dieting for a week with the menu of the third option, a month to "rest", then 5 days on the second, and after another month run to the first option of the diet.

| Options for apple weight loss | Menu for day |
| --- | --- |
| 1 | Baked apples in any quantity + water (1.5-2 liters). |
| 2 | Baked fruits (1 kg) + buttermilk (yogurt) with a low percentage of fat (1 l) + water (1 l). |
| 3 | Breakfast: vegetables (boiled), chicken fillet, croutons, for lunch and dinner: apples and water. |

For baking, choose only ripe, strong fruits, without rot, visible damage. The process should be carried out according to the following technology:

1. Wash, dry the fruit, remove the core.
2. Place in a baking dish, cook in an oven preheated to 180 ° C for about 30 minutes. The fruits should soften and acquire a golden color.
3. Optionally, you can cut the fruit into slices, spread on a baking sheet, sprinkle with a little water, and bake for a quarter of an hour.

**Diet Recipes**

The diet of apple weight loss methods is meager, so many people feel hungry. To make it easier to follow the diet and not break off halfway, it is sometimes allowed to indulge yourself with treats, for example, a pie or fruit baked with cottage cheese. The main thing is to remember that you do not need to do this every day, but once during the entire period of losing weight. Otherwise, you won't be able to lose those extra pounds.

**Baked apples with cottage cheese**

Baked fruits contain more fiber than raw ones, so they are healthier for weight loss and must be present in the diet menu. This recipe requires cottage cheese, it should be used with a minimum percentage of fat. You can eat baked fruits with a filling both hot and cold, and it is recommended to serve it sprinkled with nut crumbs.

Ingredients:

- apples (sour varieties) - 3 pcs.;
- cottage cheese - 0.3 kg;
- egg - 1 pc .;
- honey - 1 tsp;
- vanillin, cinnamon.

Cooking method:

1. Wash the fruits, cut out the core, leaving the bottom.
2. Combine the rest of the ingredients, beat with a whisk.
3. Fill the apples with the curd mass, put on a baking sheet.
4. Bake in the oven for 20-30 minutes at 150-180 °C.

**Flourless oat-apple pie**

For a variety of apple menu for dessert, you can bake a delicious, aromatic oatmeal pie. The dish is dietary because it does not contain sugar and flour, which are present in conventional baking recipes. Stevia acts as a sweetener for the treat and three types of bran are used as a thickener for the dough. This apple-oatmeal pie is a dietary version of the well-known charlotte.

Ingredients:

- apples (sour varieties) - 5 pcs .;
- egg white - 3 pcs.;
- buttermilk (1%) - 0.3 l;
- water - 0.2 l;
- stevia (honey), bran (oat) - 1 tbsp. 1 .;
- bran (rye and wheat) - 3 tbsp. 1 .;
- vanillin, cinnamon.

Cooking Method:

1. Beat the proteins with a whisk, mixer or blender until a thick foam, melt the honey.
2. Stir buttermilk with water, soda, vanilla and bran. Add honey, protein mass, mix again and let it brew for a quarter of an hour.
3. Wash the fruit, peel, chop finely, put it on the bottom of a baking dish. Sprinkle with cinnamon and pour the dough on top.
4. Bake the apple pie for 30-40 minutes at 180-200 ° C.

## Pros and cons

Any weight loss system has a number of advantages and disadvantages, and apple is no exception:

| Pros | Cons |
| --- | --- |
| <ul><li>Lowering blood cholesterol levels as a result of the systematic consumption of fruits.</li><li>Improving liver function due to the chlorogenic acid contained in fruits.</li><li>Elimination of harmful substances, breakdown of fat cells, which is facilitated by pectin.</li><li>Relief of constipation thanks to the mild laxative effect of fruits.</li><li>Decreased cravings for smoking.</li></ul> | <ul><li>The occurrence of nausea, dizziness, weakness as a result of a lack of protein and fat in the diet.</li><li>The likelihood of seizures, a malfunction of the digestive system due to a poor apple diet.</li><li>The occurrence of flatulence, bloating due to the large amount of fiber.</li></ul> |

# The Soup diet

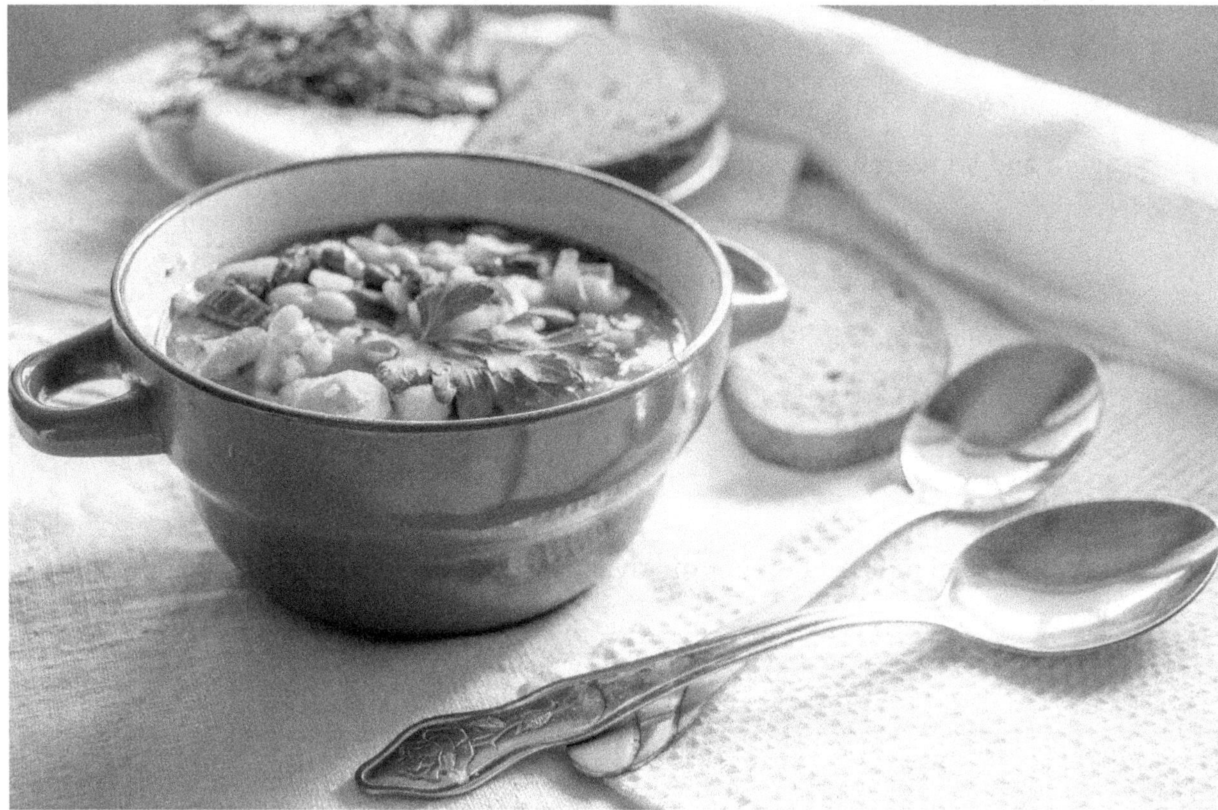

## Soup diet for weight loss

There are many options for effective diets, and one of them is soup diet. The popularity of this method of losing weight is explained simply - liquid food is easier to digest, while it can contain the entire spectrum of essential nutrients. In addition, soup is a good way to normalize digestion, replenish fluid reserves, and simply enjoy a delicious and aromatic dish.

## Benefits

- content of fiber in the broth of vegetables helps to cleanse the body of toxins, normalize digestion, and avoid constipation;
- lean meat broth contains protein, which is ideal for strengthening the body after a long illness;
- the soup warms, nourishes, restores the body's water balance;
- cooking retains a maximum of useful substances in the ingredients;
- soup is easier to fill and has fewer calories than the same volume of the second course.

**Calorie content and nutritional value**

Energy properties strongly depend on the recipe for the first course. The least high-calorie option is on water with the addition of vegetables and herbs. If the ingredients have not been fried, and there are no potatoes, the nutritional value of the broth will be only 20 kilocalories per 100 ml. If you add meat, potatoes, use vegetable oil for frying the dressing, the calorie content can reach 70 kilocalories.

## Rules and principles

The diet for weight loss with soups is low-calorie. At the same time, losing weight will not feel hungry, since the thick vegetable broth saturates well. The rules of the soup diet for weight loss:

- traditional soup diet lasts 7 days, but you can lose a little weight within 3-5 days;
- you can eat soup every 1.5 - 2 hours, but portions should be no more than 250 ml, so as not to stretch the walls of the stomach;
- you need to drink plain water between meals;
- you can combine with the main course foods that force to weight loss - pineapples (contain bromelain - a substance that "kills" fat), avocados, apples, raw vegetables;
- It is better to use vegetable broth without bread, or use whole grain breads or crackers.

## How to make a soup for weight loss

There are many recipes for making dietary soups. At the same time, the basic principles remain unchanged:

- no meat broth is used for cooking, although separately boiled meat or fish can be added to the broth;
- dieting soups should not be heavily salted, it is better to use spices;
- the main component of the broth is celery - different parts of the plant are used;
- you can cook soup according to family recipes, adding peas, soy, lentils, beans, which contain substances - fat blockers that prevent the formation of deposits;
- the broth should be cooked under the lid and no more than 20 minutes - this will help preserve vitamins;
- it is advisable to put the ingredients in boiling water.

## List of permitted foods

You can add not only vegetables, but other foods as well. Together with the broth, you can eat raw vegetables, breads, and fruits. Allowed foods include:

- squash;
- cabbage - white cabbage, cauliflower, broccoli;
- cow peas;
- artichokes;
- celery;
- green fresh peas;
- carrot;
- onions (onions, green, leek);
- beet;
- pumpkin;
- greens - spinach, dill, parsley, arugula;
- fruits - apples, pineapple, avocado;
- legumes - peas, chickpeas, lentils, beans;
- fermented milk products with a fat content of 0-1.5% - cottage cheese, yogurt, cheese;
- boiled lean meat, fish, seafood (shrimp, mussels, seafood cocktail);
- cereals - buckwheat, wild rice, wheat, barley, corn;
- eggs;
- mushrooms - champignons, oyster mushrooms, chanterelles, porcini.

## Prohibited foods

Separately, it should be said about the foods that it is advisable not to use in the menu.

Prohibited:

- fatty types of meat (pork ribs, beef, duck);
- fruits with a high glycemic index (bananas, grapes);
- animal fats (lard, lard, butter);
- smoked meats (balyk, bacon, etc.);
- sausages, sausages;
- potatoes (or use in limited quantities);

- sweets and pastries;

- home preparations, conservation;

- sweet carbonated drinks;

- sauces;

- alcohol.

## Classic soup diet for weight loss for 7 days

The weekly method of losing weight with soups is the use of not only the main dish, but also other products. For a day, you can cook 1200-1500 ml of soup, which you can eat in 5-6 receptions, and between meals you can eat vegetables, fruits, meat or dairy products. Classic fat-burning diet - 1.5 liters of soup and additives:

- 1, 6 and 7 days: 1000-1500 g of fresh vegetables;

- Day 2: 1000-1500 g of fruit;

- Day 3: vegetables and fruits (1000-1500 g);

- Day 4: 500 g of lean meat - boiled or steamed;

- Day 5: a glass of buttermilk and two apples.

## Advantages and Disadvantages

The popular and affordable soup diet for weight loss has many advantage:

- Efficiency. If you follow the recommendations of the technique, you can lose from 8 to 15 kg for the entire course.

- Budgetary. Such a diet will not burden the family budget, because cooking lunch and dinner does not require expensive ingredients;

- Benefits for digestion. A large amount of fiber helps the onionel function.

- Relative harmlessness. If, together with a dietary broth, you consume protein, fermented milk products, cereals - a weekly calorie restriction is safe for the body.

- Vegetable broth with celery lowers cholesterol, cleanses blood vessels, helps with hypertension.

- Prevention of colds. A hot soup after a winter walk will help warm up, strengthen the immune system due to vitamins.

- You won't have to starve. The soup with vegetables has low of calories, and  fills the stomach well.

The method of losing weight with liquid meals is not suitable for everyone. The food system has disadvantages:

- It is more convenient to eat first courses in specially equipped places - at home, in a cafe. If work is associated with movement around the city or the office regime does not contribute to regular absences, the diet will be a burden.
- One serving is low in calories, but even less in minerals. Many experts recommend taking a complex of trace elements during the period of weight loss.
- Fat deficiency is not the best way for mental performance.

## Diet options

There are several methods of losing weight on soups - they differ in the products used, in duration. On average, the diet can last anywhere from one day to two weeks. To choose a suitable and comfortable variety, it is worth considering your habits and body characteristics. You can create a diet according to your own preferences, taking the best from each version of the diet.

## The Finnish diet

Method, developed by Finnish nutritionists, allows you to lose 2-4 kg per week. It is possible to adhere to such a diet for longer - diet is balanced, it has everything that is necessary for the normal functioning of the body. Cons - the main course can get bored in a week. The soup is cooked simply - you need to boil carrots, parsley and celery root, white cabbage, cauliflower, garlic for half an hour, chop with a blender, add tomato juice, boil and sprinkle with herbs. Soup-puree is supplemented with the following dishes:

- porridge on the water (sources of polysaccharides);
- fermented milk products (calcium, proteins, digestion aid);
- lean meat, fish, seafood (pure protein);
- raw vegetables and fruits (dietary fiber, vitamins, trace elements).

You can eat 400-600 ml of the main course per day, organize the rest of the meal at your own discretion from the permitted products. Sample diet for the day:

- Breakfast: portion of the main course (200 ml).
- Second breakfast: oatmeal in water with honey, an apple.
- Lunch: main course, steamed chicken, raw vegetables.
- Afternoon snack: yogurt, orange, apple.
- Dinner: stewed vegetables, a glass of buttermilk.

## Diet of the Mayo Clinic

American specialists in the middle of the last century have developed their own system of weight loss on plant fibers. The Mayo Diet is based on the soup with celery, carrots, onions, tomatoes and herbs, which is able to "cleanse" the body. In addition to vegetable broth, wild rice, vegetables, lean meat, fruits are allowed. The advantages of the diet are that you can lose 5-6 kg in a week, and the disadvantage is low calorie content. Dieting for more than a week is not worth it, so as not to provoke health problems. Vegetable broth must be eaten 5-6 times a day, supplementing the meal with permitted products:

- 1 day: fruit - 1000 g;
- Day 2: fresh vegetables - 1000 g;
- Day 3: vegetables and fruits - 1000 g;
- Day 4: 400 g of boiled meat (veal or chicken), 300 g of vegetables;
- Day 5: fruits (oranges and bananas);
- Day 6: 400 g of steamed meat, 300 g of green vegetables;
- Day 7: 300 g of wild rice, vegetables and fruits (500 g).

## Fasting Day

Not everyone is willing to eat a soup diet for a week or more to get leaner. A soft way to lose weight a little (0.5 - 1.5 kg) can be a fasting day. You need to prepare 1-1.5 liters of the main course (according to the Finnish recipe or the Mayo Clinic) and eat it during the day without adding anything. To enhance the effect, do not salt, but drink water between meals. The advantages of a fasting day are short duration. Cons - it is better to plan unloading on the weekend, since such a set of products with water has a diuretic effect.

## Mono-diet for 3 days

You can lose 3-4 kilograms in three days if you sit on a mono-diet. The technique allows you to consume 1-1.2 liters of soup (vegetable, buckwheat, pea, chicken) per day, which should include celery root and drink at least 2 liters of water. As a variety, it is allowed to eat 1-2 apples a day. Pros - fast and confident weight loss, cons - severe dietary restrictions can stress the body. Headaches, irritability and sleep disturbances are possible.

## Recipes for dietary soups for weight loss

In order not to think about what to cook for breakfast or lunch during a diet, you can use ready-made recipes for dietary dishes. Slimming soups can be made from a variety of foods, or vegetables can be combined by color. You can enhance the taste of the dish with a mixture of spices, garlic and red pepper. Use greens at the end to preserve the flavor.

**Bonn Soup**

- Time: 30 minutes.
- Servings: 10.
- Calorie content: 20 kcal per 100 g.
- Cuisine: German.
- Difficulty: Medium.
- Purpose: for weight loss.

A delicious and appetizing famous Bonn soup will help you lose weight with pleasure - Hollywood actress Renee Zellweger lost weight on it. This dish "works" like a brush - cleanses the intestines and makes smooth muscles work more actively. The Bonn recipe should be used when you need to get rid of edema, to make your skin healthier.

**Ingredients**

- white cabbage - 200 g;
- celery root and leaves - 100 g;
- Bulgarian pepper - 100 g;
- onion - 1 head;
- tomatoes - 3 pcs.;
- water - 1.2 l;
- Basil, thyme, salt.

**Cooking method:**

1. Chop cabbage, celery root, pepper and onion and toss into a saucepan with boiling water.
2. Boil over low heat for 15 minutes.
3. During this time, peel the tomatoes, cut into cubes. Grind the herbs.
4. Pour tomatoes and herbs into the boiling broth, add salt and spices.
5. Boil for another 5 minutes under the lid, let it brew. Serve hot.

**Celery soup**

- Time: 35 minutes.
- Servings: 8.
- Calorie content: 16 kcal per 100 g.
- Cuisine: Italian.
- Difficulty: Medium.
- Purpose: for weight loss.

Celery soup is the gold standard for weight loss. This root perfectly cleans the intestines. In this case, all parts of the plant are used - the root, stem and leaves. Parsley root and chopped herbs work well with this component. Carrots contain pectin, which normalizes digestion, and if potatoes are added to the dish, the calorie content will increase slightly, but the taste will become softer.

**Ingredients**

- root, stem, celery leaves - 300 g;
- onion - 1 head;
- carrots - 1 pc.;
- parsley root - 50 g;
- water - 1.2 l;
- spices and salt.

**Cooking method**

1. Bring water to a boil.
2. Add chopped vegetables - onions, carrots, parsley, celery root and stalk.
3. Cook covered over low heat for 15 minutes.
4. Add chopped celery leaves, spices and salt.
5. Cover and let it brew for 10 minutes.

**Cream Soup**

- Time: 35 minutes.
- Servings: 8.
- Calorie content: 22 kcal per 100 g.
- Cuisine: French.
- Difficulty: Medium.

- Purpose: for weight loss.

A delicate puree soup served in top restaurants, this dish has a silky, flowing texture and green color through the use of watercress. You can cook it for the whole family, and everyone can add a spoonful of sour cream to a plate. This dish contains celery, but only the stem is used - a fragrant and extremely useful component.

**Ingredients**

- stalked celery - 100 g;
- watercress - 200 g;
- leeks - 1 stalk;
- potatoes - 1 pc.;
- olive oil - 1 tablespoon;
- nutmeg - a pinch;
- garlic - 2 cloves.

**Cooking method:**

1. Heat a cast iron saucepan, pour olive oil on the bottom.
2. Cut the leeks into rings, press the garlic with the flat side of a knife. Fry onions and garlic for 5 minutes.
3. Bring the water to a boil in a separate onionl, pour over the onion and garlic.
4. Cut potatoes and celery stalks into cubes or slices, add to the broth.
5. Cook over low heat for 10 minutes.
6. Cut the watercress, pour into a saucepan, season with salt, add nutmeg.
7. Boil for another 5 minutes.
8. Cool slightly and grind the broth with vegetables through a sieve or beat with a blender.

**Contraindications**

Dieting with a soup diet permitted  only after consulting a doctor. The main contraindications are as follows:

- Pregnancy. The impact on the fetus of such a diet can be unpredictable.
- Women during lactation - the use of a decoction with celery can cause diarrhea in the baby.

- Disorders of the digestive tract. Some diseases of the digestive tract when eating food can cause bloating, colic.
- Anemia. Micronutrient deficiencies with dietary restrictions will exacerbate the problem.
- Kidney disease. Celery crushes kidney stones, and its decoction has a diuretic effect. All this in combination can provoke the exit of calculi.
- Phlebeurysm. Celery dilates blood vessels, which can be dangerous in case of venous pathologies.
- Hypotension and cardiovascular disease - vegetable decoctions reduce blood pressure.
- A tendency to diarrhea, flatulence.

## What to do in case of a breakdown

In different cases, nutritionists recommend different attitudes towards a breakdown of the diet. In this case, one should act according to the following scheme:

- Assess the damage. If the regime has been violated only once, there will be no big harm to the figure - small indulgences can speed up the metabolism and proceed losing weight.
- If you had to break loose at the festive table, you should try to burn the calories gained through physical activity - cycling, jogging, strength exercises.
- Be prepared to increase the duration of the diet.

## How to get out of the diet

It is important not only to achieve your goal, but also to stabilize your weight. This is achieved by gradual adaptation to the usual diet after the end of the diet. It is advisable to restore the diet habitual for the body within two weeks. In the first three days, it is recommended to replace one of the meals with a more high-calorie one, but not to increase the portion. For the next three to four days, continue to consume the base dish, but only once a day. Further, gradually increase the energy value of products, gradually abandoning the soup with celery.

# The Zucchini diet

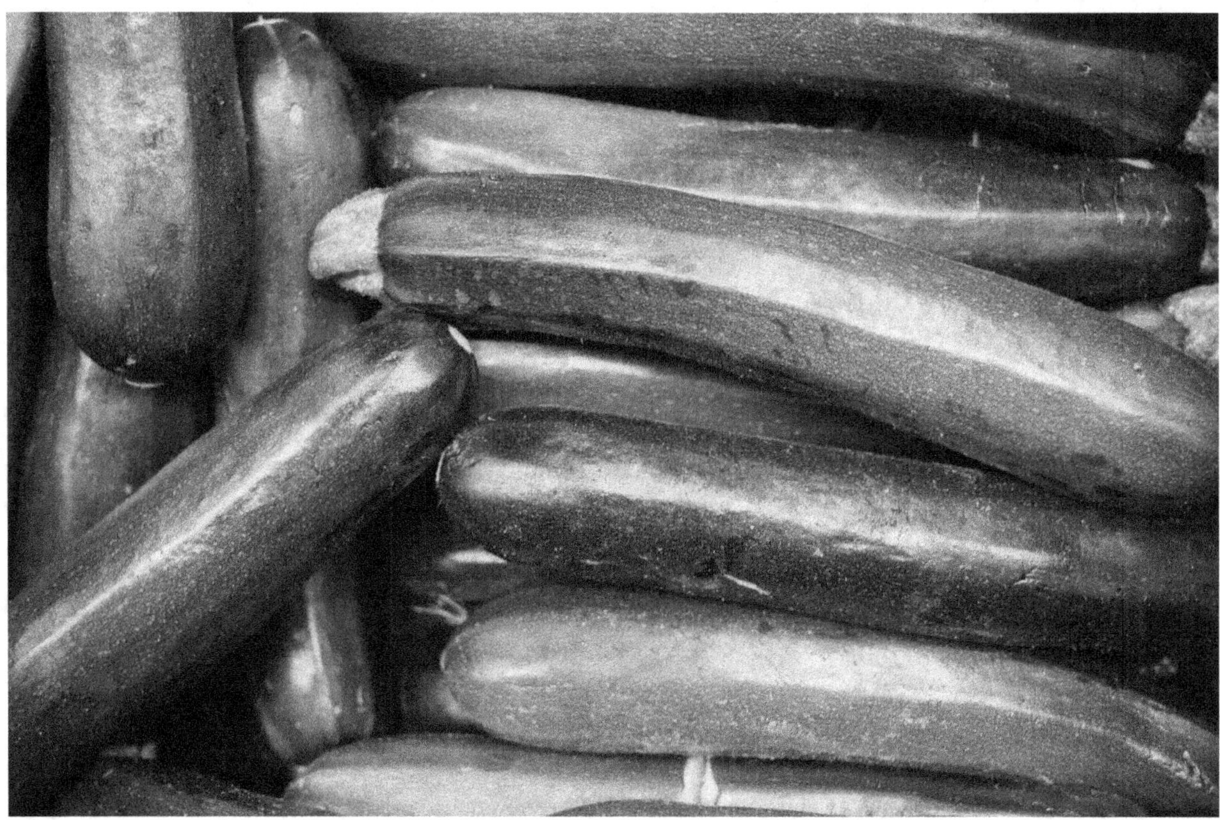

You can hear many positive reviews about the zucchini-based diet menu for weight loss, or the zucchini diet. An unpretentious vegetable, which is not difficult to grow in the country, in summer and autumn can become a real boon for those who want to improve their body health, remove 5-10 kilograms of excess weight. It goes well with other dietary products and allows you to prepare a wide variety of delicious, low-calorie meals.

## What are the benefits of zucchini for the body?

 Diet on zucchini removes toxins from the body, accelerates the blood purification process, activates the urinary system, reduces water, salt, normalizes heart function, lowers cholesterol, and increases immunity. Its observance guarantees the intake of vitamins and minerals necessary for a person for normal life, among which are vitamins A, E, C, B, PP, potassium, calcium, magnesium, iron, carotene, etc. Zucchini does not cause allergies, is indicated for sugar diabetes, cardiovascular diseases, gastritis.

## Zucchini for weight loss

The first stage of weight loss is the normalization of the water-salt body balance. Zucchini juice has diuretic properties, helping the fastest elimination of water and salt from the body. With its help, you can not only get rid of extra pounds, but also cure serious diseases arising from excess water content - for example, cardiac edema (respectively, as an adjunct to drug therapy).

Any method of losing weight involves cleansing the intestines. Regular consumption of 500 g of zucchini within a week will significantly improve the peristalsis of the gastrointestinal tract, normalize metabolism, and remove toxins accumulated in the body. Vegetables do not irritate the gastric and intestinal mucosa, their effect is mild and protective.

## Zucchini diet for quick weight loss

The low calorie content of this vegetable crop - 100 g contains only 20 kcal - makes it an excellent basis for unloading nutrition. You can eat 1.5 kg daily without the risk of gaining weight. The dietary menu, which is based on dishes from zucchini, should be adhered to for a short time - from 3 to 14 days, depending on the expected effect. The essence of unloading comes down to use of a vegetable in different heat treatment options. The dishes are light, you can eat a lot of them, so the diet is easily tolerated.

## Benefits of the diet

Zucchini fits well with a large amount of low-calorie foods, there are many recipes for cooking meals and drinks with this vegetable. So the diet menu can be varied. The main ingredient has a calming effect on ingestion, does not cause irritation, side effects, therefore the squash diet shows good results within a week after its start. In addition, many useful substances enter the body during the diet.

## Rules

The basic rules to be followed by dieters require a combination of a low-calorie squash menu while replenishing the "losses" resulting from the rejection of the usual food. The laudable desire to get rid of a few extra pounds should not be accompanied by a deficiency of nutrients in the body. It is worth following these recommendations:

- cook without oil and fat, otherwise the calorie content of the dishes greatly increases;
- you need to cook a vegetable with a peel, it contains the most vitamins and minerals;
- add other vegetables, fruits, low-calorie protein products to dishes;
- during a diet, you must drink at least 2 liters of water per day;
- give up alcohol, potatoes, sweets, pastries, smoked meats, pickles;
- you need to eat often, in small portions;
- start taking multivitamins with minerals to replenish the body's losses.

## Contraindications

During unloading, water and minerals are excreted from the body, therefore it is contraindicated for pregnant women, adolescents during puberty and everyone for whom a deficiency of nutrients may be critical. On the other hand, with zucchini, a lot of potassium is launched into the body. It can be harmful for chronic diseases of the urinary system. In its raw form, zucchini is prohibited for use who suffering from gastritis.

## Zucchini diet menu

You can cook dishes in different ways: bake, stew, cook as an independent dish with the addition of onions, tomatoes, bell peppers, herbs, and as a component of complex dishes in combination with low-fat fish, eggs, poultry, cottage cheese, yogurt. When drawing up the menu, it should be borne in mind that the basis of vegetable soups, salads, stews, caviar, pancakes, casseroles, juices, etc. should be zucchini, its content in the dish should be at least 50%.

**An approximate diet menu may be as follows:**

## For 3 days

|  | breakfast | lunch | dinner |
|---|---|---|---|
| **1 day** | vegetable casserole with cottage cheese, green tea | puree soup with carrots and celery, boiled chicken, rosehip broth | vegetables baked in foil, buttermilk |
| **2 day** | vegetable pancakes, green tea | fish with a vegetable stew garnish, water | baked vegetables stuffed with cottage cheese, buttermilk |
| **3 day** | boiled egg, vegetable juice | soup with mushrooms and onions, boiled beef, any juice | vegetable stew, buttermilk |

## For 7 days

|  | Breakfast | Lunch | Dinner |
|---|---|---|---|
| **4 day** | omelet with addition vegetables, green tea | puree soup with mushrooms and carrots, boiled chicken, rosehip broth; | vegetable caviar, buttermilk |
| **5 day** | vegetable pancakes, green tea | fish, vegetable stew with zucchini, water | vegetables baked with mushroom filling, buttermilk |
| **6 day** | boiled egg, vegetable juice from raw zucchini | soup with carrots and onions, boiled beef, vegetable juice | vegetable stew, buttermilk |
| **Day 7** | zucchini pancakes, green tea | chicken broth, boiled beef, vegetable stew, water | vegetables baked with cottage cheese, yogurt |

**For 14 days**

|  | breakfast | lunch | dinner |
|---|---|---|---|
| **8 day** | vegetable salad with cucumber, bell pepper and yogurt; | cream soup with mushrooms and onions, boiled beef, water | vegetable caviar, buttermilk |
| **9 day** | salad with apple, boiled chicken, olive oil | boiled fish, boiled rice with stewed vegetables, water | baked vegetables stuffed with mushrooms, buttermilk |
| **10 day** | omelet with the addition of zucchini, green tea | boiled chicken, vegetable stew, water | vegetable caviar, buttermilk |
| **11 day** | vegetable casserole, green tea | chicken broth, boiled beef, vegetable stew, rosehip broth | vegetables baked with cottage cheese, buttermilk |
| **12 day** | vegetable pancakes, rosehip broth | soup - mashed potatoes with the addition of carrots and celery, boiled chicken, squash caviar, water | vegetables baked in foil, buttermilk |
| **day 13** | vegetable pancakes, green tea | puree soup with mushrooms and onions, stewed fish, vegetable salad, water | vegetable caviar, buttermilk |
| **day 14** | rice porridge with vegetables,broth | boiled chicken, vegetable stew,water | squash casserole, buttermilk |

**Diet on mashed zucchini**

Judging by the reviews, mashed zucchini is an ideal dish for weight loss. Seven-day squash unloading will help get rid of 2-4 kg of excess weight. Mashed zucchini with a diet is prepared as follows: the zucchini is baked in the oven, the rest of the vegetables - onions, carrots, tomatoes - are stewed separately.

Then the ingredients must be mixed in a blender, the finished product must be put in jars. The diet may look like this:

|  | **Breakfast** | **Lunch** | **Dinner** |
|---|---|---|---|
| **1-7 days** | Low-fat cottage cheese and squash caviar, green tea | Boiled chicken breast, squash caviar, rosehip broth | Boiled fish, squash caviar, buttermilk |

# The Choco diet

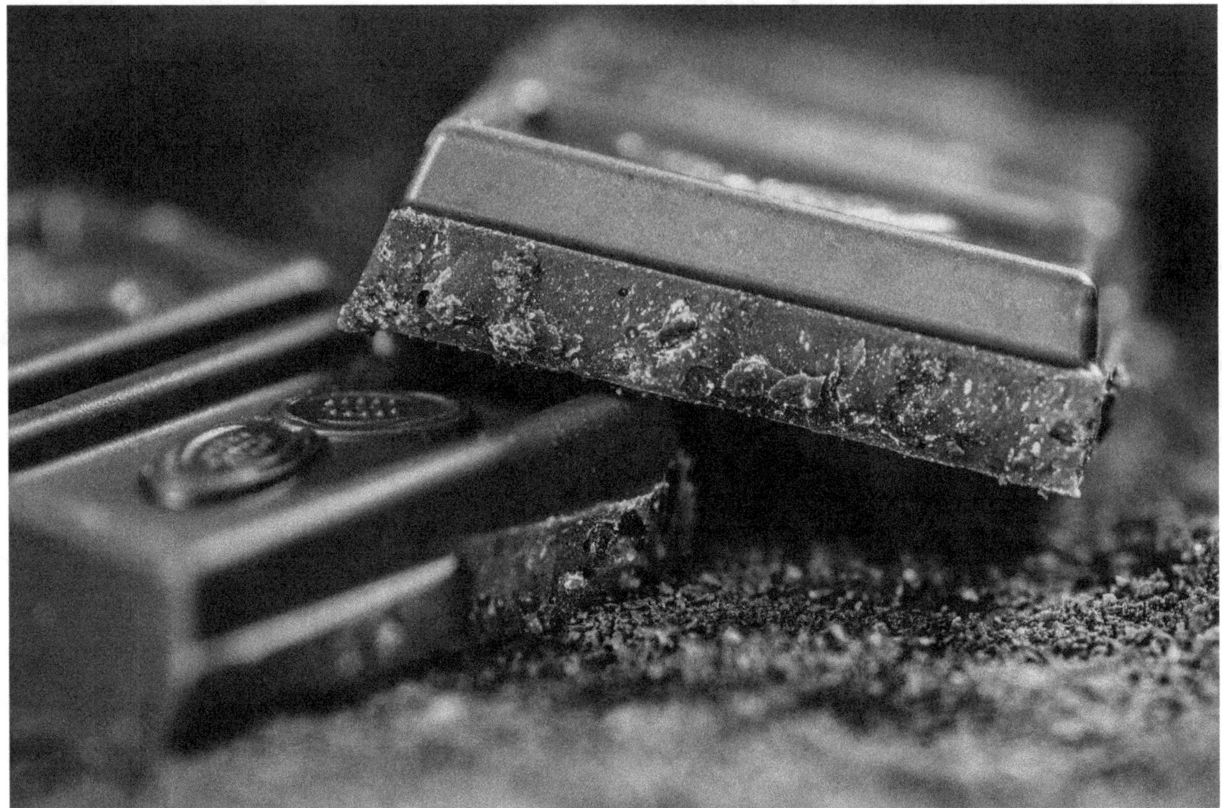

It takes tremendous willpower to lose those extra pounds, especially for those who cannot imagine their life without sweets and chocolate. Losing weight with a choko-diet will be that lifesaver when you can't refuse sweets and coffee, it will give excellent results in just a week, and the menu can be made in such a way that the lost kilograms do not return. Subject to all conditions, up to 7 kilograms are dropped. However, you need to understand that this diet is very tough, so if you have health problems, it is better to refuse it.

## What is the choko-diet?

The chocolate diet for weight loss is featured in two options: the classic diet and the drinking chocolate diet. The difference is that in the first case, to combat excess weight, several pieces of chocolate are eaten during the day, but the total weight is no more than 100 g, everything is washed down with coffee without sugar. You can supplement the diet with fresh and boiled vegetables, durum wheat pasta.

Drinking a chocolate diet also gives an excellent result and can take away 6-7 kg. It is allowed not to drink chocolate with black coffee. Instead, you can drink cocoa, hot chocolate (5-6 cups per day). There is no difference, hot or cold drink. However, it must be remembered that cold food requires more energy for its absorption, and it can be obtained from warm food. The most important condition is: "NO SUGAR!"

**Basic rules**

A diet on chocolate presupposes compliance with some rules, but the most important rule is constant physical activities. The rules will help you lose more pounds without harming the body:

1. Choose dark chocolate.
2. A 100 g bar is divided into three parts, eaten in 3 doses, washed down with black coffee.
3. When drinking liquid, observe the drinking regime: at least 1.5 liters of water.
4. Hot chocolate, cocoa, cocktails are allowed.
5. In order not to starve oneself, vegetables rich in vitamins are added to the menu.
6. Durum wheat pasta is allowed.
7. It is forbidden to dilute drinks with sugar, eat fried food, dilute vegetable salads with oil. You can not eat fruits, juices from them. Carbonated and alcoholic drinks are excluded.


**What Chocolates You Can Eat**

With a chocolate diet, the most important rule is to choose the basic product. All nutritionists agree on one thing: dark chocolate has a positive effect on weight loss. This is explained by the fact that this product has a low glycemic index. It's very good when meals are 30 minutes after eating dark chocolate: it reduces appetite, speeds up metabolism, which leads to a normal weight of a person.


**Diet menu**

In order to painlessly dieting on a low-calorie course, it is important to create a balanced menu. The chocolate method is based on a strict diet: there are many restrictions. Therefore, it is important to think over your diet so that not only is weight loss, but also the stomach works properly. It is not enough to reduce the daily caloric intake, it is necessary to ensure that the necessary trace elements and vitamins for energy production are obtained. This is possible due to the addition of vegetables to the diet.

When it comes to meals, breakfast, lunch, and dinner are very similar, with dark chocolate, coffee, or a drinking cocktail drink selected for the main meal. If there are other permitted products on the menu, then a bar of chocolate, divided into three parts, is eaten 30 minutes before meals. After a couple of hours after eating, you can drink water, green tea. Drinking water is mandatory.

**3 days**

This type of chocolate diet lasts for three days. After the end, it is imperative to take a break and get out of it very slowly and carefully. Choco-diet is suitable for those who urgently need to lose three kilograms, as happens before important events.

**Main requirements:**

1. Eaten only 100 g of chocolate a day.
2. The bar can be cut into three pieces or eaten in one go. Everything is washed down with black coffee.
3. Green tea is acceptable. Other drinks are prohibited.
4. Drink plenty of clean, non-carbonated water between meals.
5. Avoiding alcohol.

The complexity of such a mono-diet is in strict restrictions. The slimming effect is achieved by avoiding salt and sugar. After three days, the result is clearly visible also due to the fact that excess fluid is removed from the body. The disadvantage of such a diet is that protein and other nutrients do not come with food. This can negatively affect the condition of the skin and hair.

**7 days**

The authors of the method call it Italian chocolate diet because it was invented by Italian nutritionists. A beautiful name immediately attracts attention. The 7-day chocolate diet involves consuming 30 g of dark chocolate per day. The plus is that during this period, you can eat other foods, for example, pasta, sauces, low-fat gravies. Lemon juice or low-fat yogurt is used as a salad dressing; you cannot dress with vegetable or olive oil. The menu includes vegetables and fruits, except for grapes, bananas and potatoes. Be sure to drink water.

The diet for 7 days allows the use of vitamins with increased fatigue. It is important to combine foods correctly. The sample menu is as follows:

- breakfast: salad, oatmeal porridge;
- 2nd breakfast: 10 g of dark chocolate and 1 fruit;
- lunch: pasta and salad dressed with lemon juice;
- afternoon snack: 10 g of dark chocolate and 1 fruit;
- dinner: tomato paste, vegetable salad or boiled vegetables;
- 2nd dinner: 10 g of dark chocolate.

**7 Days drinking diet**

The drinking diet is distinguished by the consumption of liquid chocolate, cocoa, or chocolate shakes. To start the process of losing weight, you must drink at least 6 cups of a drink with a volume of 200 ml per day. In addition, you should drink about two liters of water. The chocolate drink should be warm. After 7 days, the weight can decrease by 6-7 kg.

There are two types of drinking diet. The first is to use only cocoa or a liquid chocolate drink (if desired, you can dilute with low-fat milk), the second - dark chocolate, green tea or coffee. To reduce the calorie content, it is recommended to dilute the liquid drink with water (ratio: 1 to 1). Cocoa is prepared with water and milk. The powder is added to taste, but the optimal amount: for 1 liter of liquid (ordinary water, mixture or skim milk) 3 tablespoons.

This type of diet is considered the safest and easiest. On Juliette Kellow's chocolate diet, you can easily remove up to 4 kg per week without much difficulty. The best part is the menu is balanced, which does not give you a feeling of hunger. Basic requirements:

- drink at least 6 glasses of water;
- eat 3 times a day, each time eating a chocolate bar in any form, even a candy will do;
- snacks with chocolate, weight - up to 30 g;
- skim milk is allowed - up to 300 ml;
- salads are seasoned with low-fat, sugar-free yogurt.

**Exit from the chocolate diet**

The return to normal nutrition should be very careful. In order not to gain weight again, you need to follow certain rules. It is recommended:

1. On the first day, drink juices or fresh juices without sugar.
2. Do not overuse salt.
3. For the next three days, add boiled vegetables to the diet. It is best to use cabbage.
4. Introduce several new products daily: fish, buckwheat porridge, boiled breast, rice.

**Contraindications**

It is clear that the diet is designed for people who find it very difficult to refuse sweets. However, before deciding to use it, you need to find out if there are any contraindications. Chocolate is a prohibited food for many diseases, so it is important to know for sure whether diet will be beneficial. It is quite possible that other problems will appear with the lost kilograms, which will take much longer to solve.

**Who can and to whom is the chocolate technique contraindicated?**

 Before starting to lose weight, it is important to examine the liver, kidneys, gastrointestinal tract, heart. It is forbidden to use diets for:

- liver diseases;
- hypertension;
- diseases of the cardiovascular system;
- diabetes mellitus;
- allergies to chocolate;

# The Banana diet

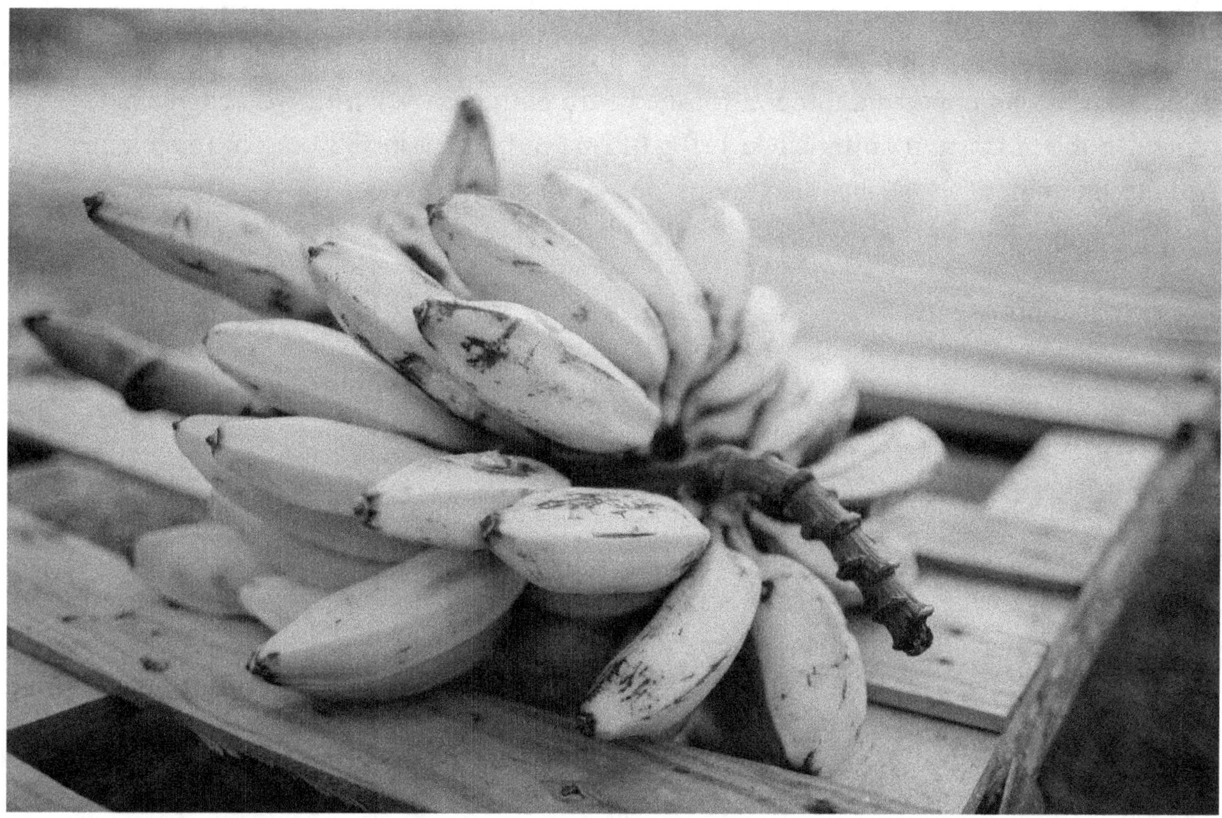

Most weight loss diets deny the use of bananas because it is believed that this fruit is not suitable for a diet aimed at losing weight due to its high calorie content. But the existence of a banana diet  doubts this claim. Who is wrong - people who suggest losing weight with bananas, or opponents of it used in the process of creating a slender body?

## Is it possible to lose weight on bananas?

The reason why experts doubt about banana weight loss schemes is the high calorie content of the main product: 100 g contains 89 kcal (according to some sources - 95 kcal), 21.8 g of carbohydrates and a large amount of sugar. It is the reason why  the banana diet is not the best choice for those who want to lose weight,according to nutritionists. Against the large amount of sugar, this fruit provokes an insulin jump, which then causes a new attack of hunger.

However:

- if the diet involves a fasting day, weight will be lost due to a strong decrease in daily calorie intake;
- Bananas, like other plant foods, launched into mono diets, help cleanse the body, which also leads to weight loss, but  will not improve the quality of the body.

## Useful properties and consist of bananas

The entire plant group, even with a considerable calorie content, contains natural sugar. It has a lot of valuable qualities. So bananas can be called the biggest holders for the content of potassium - an important mineral for the heart: eating only 1 fruit, you can easily replenish the potassium norm, since 100 g of ripe pulp contains 358 mg of this element. Among the minerals, one can also highlight:

- calcium;
- phosphorus;
- iron;
- magnesium (indirectly helps metabolism).

Banana is an excellent source of energy in part due to its high glycemic index (over 70 units) and is high in starch. Banana is a good product for people suffering from poor functioning of the gastrointestinal tract, gastritis, diarrhea, however, it is not allowed to take a tough banana weight loss scheme with such problems.

## Diet on bananas

The authorship of such an unusual body shaping technique is attributed to British nutritionist Jane Griffin, who was one of the first to tell how to use banana fruits for weight loss - they were previously considered an anti-dietary product. The system is soft, but you can stick to its rules for no longer than a week. The approximate weight loss is 6 kg, but the exact figure can only be determined when the initial parameters are specified. The power system has several important points:

- The day before it, you need to prepare: drink only mineral water without gas and green tea, do not eat fatty and fried foods.
- Eat all plant foods as fresh as possible.
- You cannot combine bananas with cereals on the menu: you will have to eat oatmeal separately, in a different meal.

## Indications for Use

Most people perceive figure-building diets as an enemy of health, but banana diets may even be beneficial. This is explained not only by the large amount of vitamins and valuable minerals in this fruit, but also by the high level of starch, which reduces stomach discomfort and soothes the intestines. There is a list of diseases for which such a menu will be of a therapeutic nature for a short time:

- hypoglycemia (low sugar, can manifest itself in attacks);
- chronic stomach problems - gastritis, gastroduodenitis;
- diseases of the liver and urinary system;
- disturbances in the work of the biliary tract;
- circulatory problems.

## What you can and cannot eat on a diet

Any weight loss diet is based primarily on reducing the daily calorie intake, therefore, if you create a menu, there can be no "heavy" foods in terms of calorie content and the proportion of carbohydrates. Some categories from the dairy and fermented milk groups, other fruits or vegetables are added to the main fruit. It is not excluded the use of whole grain breads, so as not to forget about complex carbohydrates at all. It is obligatory to refuse from:

- sources of sugar (not fruits, but factory sweets are meant);
- fried foods;
- fatty foods;
- meat and fish (some diets, if they are long, allow a very small portion);
- pickled and salted dishes.

## What fruits to choose for weight loss

Experts continue to argue about the degree of maturity of the main product of the banana diet: some nutritionists recommend eating green fruits (more precisely, those that have begun to turn yellow), since they contain less sugar and pectin, and the fiber in dense pulp is coarser. However, the percentage of starch that is dangerous for the figure, the degree of maturity is inversely proportional: the softer the fruit, the less of this substance in it. Unripe fruit can have a glycemic index of 42 units, so it is preferable on a diet. Banana chips shouldn't be touched.

## How to lose weight on bananas in 3 days

A short and simple technique that helps you lose 2-3 kg of excess weight involves eating fresh, dense bananas, green apples and cucumbers. These products are diuretic and known for their cleansing properties, so do your weight loss and detox on weekends. Do not forget about clean water: 1.8-2 liters must be drunk daily. The three-day diet will be structured as follows:

- breakfast - 2 bananas;
- snack - an apple;
- lunch - banana and apple;
- dinner - a cucumber.

**Banana diet for 7 days**

For those who are not afraid of difficulties, a weekly diet is suitable. For a day, 1 kg of fresh fruit is allocated (this is up to 950 kcal), 2-2.5 liters of pure water, 0.5 liters of green tea and mineral water. Only breakfast changes daily, which will be include:

1. 3 boiled quail eggs.
2. 2 oranges.
3. 2 boiled chicken eggs.
4. Grapefruit. If the day looks hungry, you can eat 300 ml of vegetable broth (no potatoes) during the day.
5. 3 boiled quail eggs.
6. 2 oranges.
7. 2 boiled chicken eggs.

**Fasting day**

The meaning of the technique is a  rejection of all other products: in a day you can eat 1 kg of banana (this is no more than 950 kcal), breaking this volume into 6-8 meals with equal intervals. In addition, it is imperative to drink a lot, mainly clean warm water, but green tea and mineral water are also allowed. Some nutritionists allow adding skim lactose-free milk to the diet - up to 0.5 liters.

**Varieties of a mono-diet**

There are a lot of options for banana diets, but mainly experts advise combining the main fruit with milk, buttermilk or cottage cheese. These schemes are the most effective and relatively satisfying, since protein is added to the starch.

The softer one is designed for 5 days, but can be reduced to 3 days. About 500 g is lost per day, but if you are overweight, a person may notice the withdrawal of 800 g. Basic rules:

- For a day, you take 350 g of fruits (3 pcs.) And 600 ml of milk without lactose and a minimum (0.5%) fat content.
- You can drink clean water in any volume.

- You need to eat 4 times a day.
- The last meal is required at 18:00.

In the strict version of the banana-milk diet, which is designed for 10 days, the menu is almost the same, and the general rules for food intake and water regime are similar. However, the proportion of milk increases to 1 liter per day, and, if necessary, you can replace low-fat buttermilk or drinking yogurt, devoid of additives. However, the latter is allowed only 0.5 liters. Fruit with a diet of 10 days is eaten in an amount of 4 pieces. (about 450 g) per day.

## Banana + Cottage Cheese for Weight Loss

The four-day strict weight loss method, suggests alternating banana and cottage cheese days, is suitable for persons who do not like to starve while losing weight. Its effectiveness overshadowed the other mono diets on this fruit, since the body does not suffer from protein deficiency. You can lose 4-5 kg in 4 days, keeping your working capacity as much as possible. The menu is organized as follows:

- Odd or banana days: in the morning banana + milk (glass), in the afternoon banana + egg (boil), in the evening banana + chicken (breast, 150 g, boil).
- Even for cottage cheese days: in the morning cottage cheese + grapefruit (100 g), in the afternoon cottage cheese + apples (200 g), the evening is similar to the morning. Cottage cheese is 5% fat.

## The Japanese

Methodology, which came from Asia, does not quite correspond to the mono-diet format, since it allows the use of third-party products, requiring only one rule to be followed - eat 1-2 raw bananas every morning. After 3-4 hours, you can have a full lunch, after which you can have an afternoon snack and dinner. After 20 hours, nothing but water is taken into the mouth. The diet lasts a week. During the day, preference is given to soft foods:

- water cereals (dairy products are prohibited);
- stewed / steamed vegetables.

## Buttermilk-banana

A simple substitute for the milk-banana diet can be a course based on low-fat buttermilk and non-thermally processed fruits. The non-thermally processed fruits are used in the amount of 6 pieces. per day, which will be about 700 g (you should not gain more than 700 kcal), and you can drink a whole liter of buttermilk - this will be 400 kcal. So your daily calorie intake will not be too underestimated, so the body will suffer minimally. The banana-buttermilk technique can be observed for up to 5 days.

**Recipes for dietary dishes**

There are a lot of ways to use banana pulp in cooking - it's launched into the dough, it's used for fruit casseroles, salads, cocktails (smoothies), cold desserts. However, when losing weight, most recipes are prohibited: nutritionists advise using this fruit mostly fresh, in protein shakes or light salads.

**Banana cocktail with buttermilk and cinnamon**

- Servings: 1 person.
- Calorie content: 264 kcal.

If you are looking for delicious and non-threatening recipes for yourself, you need to try a delicious cocktail. It consists of buttermilk (choose one that has stood for 2-3 days - not the freshest one), or skim milk, which does not contain lactose, a pinch of cinnamon and banana puree. If you wish, you can add a couple of fresh strawberries, and take a teaspoon of honey for sweetness.

Ingredients:

- banana - 120 g;
- buttermilk - 200 ml;
- honey - 1 tsp;
- cinnamon - 1 tsp

Cooking method:

1. Using a blender, make a banana puree (spin for a minute at high speed).
2. Mix with a glass of buttermilk in the same place, add honey and cinnamon. Shake up for another 20 seconds.

**Baked Bananas**

- Servings: 2 persons.
- Calorie content: 357 kcal.

**Ingredients:**

- bananas - 240 g;
- cottage cheese - 50 g;
- lemon - 1/2 pc.;
- egg white - 20 g;

- natural yogurt - 50 g;
- cinnamon - 1/2 tsp.

### Cooking method:

1. Put the sliced fruit on the bottom of the ceramic dish (take 2 - it's easier to divide the portions this way).
2. Drizzle with lemon juice.
3. Whisk the protein with yogurt and cottage cheese (preferably in briquette format), cover the banana layer.
4. Sprinkle with cinnamon, bake for 15 minutes at 200 degrees.

### How to get out of the diet

Banana weight loss schemes are classified as tough. To consolidate the result and prevent malfunctions in the gastrointestinal tract - required to conduct the correct exit. Firstly, in terms of duration, it must correspond to the duration of the diet itself: if you lost weight for 4 days, exactly the same amount you will slowly and gradually launch familiar foods. The output algorithm looks like this:

1. The first stage is the addition of vegetables and unsweetened fruits that were not used during the diet. Increase daily calorie intake by only 100-200 kcal.
2. The second stage is the return to the diet of cereals in water or milk, but without additives. Oatmeal, rice, buckwheat are desirable.
3. The third stage is the use of a small (up to 150 g per day) amount of lean meat, fish or seafood in the diet.
4. The last stage is to supplement the menu with whole grain bread, cheeses, fermented milk products, pasta, but in turn: 1 day - 1 food group.

### Contraindications and side effects

None of the options for banana deloading or even milder regimens can be used for those who suffer from diabetes, due to the high glycemic index of the main product. A similar recommendation is given in case of individual intolerance to the main fruit and the appearance of allergic reactions. During weight loss, nausea, weakness are not excluded. Some experts point out that no banana diet can be prescribed for:

- liver disease;

- problems with the bile ducts;

- exacerbated gastrointestinal diseases;

- thrombophlebitis, high blood clotting rate;

- ischemic heart disease;

- diarrhea (if combined with milk).

# Protein diets
## Meat diet

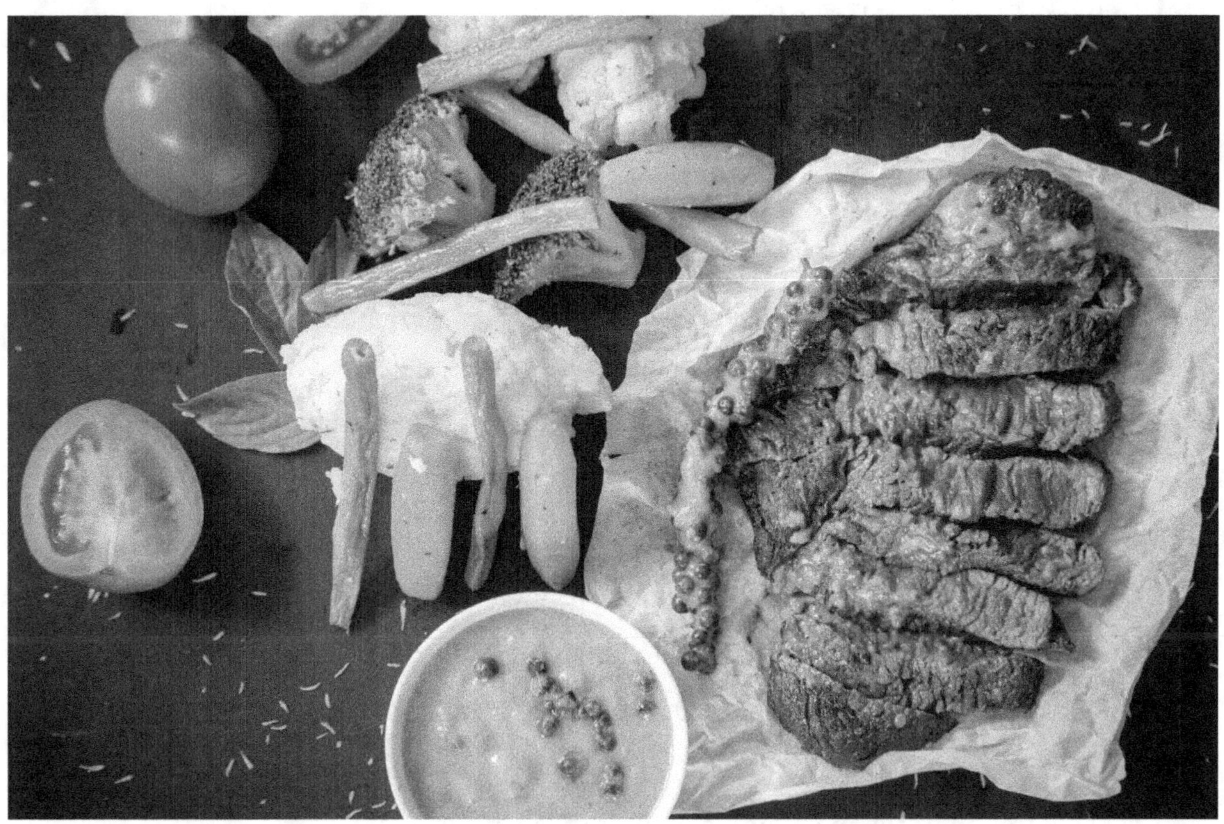

The popular diet of meat and vegetables helps to quickly lose weight without harm to health. The basis of the diet is use of predominantly low-fat meat dishes. The number of meals is determined individually, on average - from 3 to 5.

**Advantages and disadvantages of the meat diet**

The advantages:

- lack of hunger;
- quick relief from edema;
- stabilization of blood sugar levels;
- minimal loss of muscle tissue during weight loss.

The disadvantages:

- constant weakness, drowsiness;
- bad breath;
- psychological discomfort.

**Meal rules on a meat diet**

To get the maximum effect, you should follow several rules and recommendations:

1. allowed to eat any lean meat.
2. The daily amount of meat is not more than 500 grams.
3. The daily calorie content is 1600-1700 kcal.
4. Diet meat dishes should be supplemented with fresh or stewed vegetables (except for potatoes, carrots).
5. Cereals, pastries, sweets, nuts are prohibited.
6. It is necessary to refuse flour, sweet alcohol, and sauces.
7. You can supplement the meat diet with chicken or quail eggs (no more than 2 per day). Low-fat cottage cheese (2-3 times a week).
8. Limit the amount of salt to 3 g per day.
9. Before cooking meat, you need to remove fat and skin.
10. Consume 1-2 tbsp daily. of unrefined olive oil or 5 g of butter. This will help avoid disruption of the hormonal system, dry skin, hair loss.
11. Dinner - no later than 8 pm.
12. The duration of the meat diet is no more than 10 days.
13. Drink 100-200 ml of low-fat two-day buttermilk with bran daily to maintain

onionel function.


## Types of Meat Diets

All such protein diets are divided into groups according to duration, type of meat products consumed and a set of additional products. You can keep the diet from 3 to 10 days, choose one of the proposed meat options and supplement the diet with permitted foods.

Duration is determined by the amount of excess weight. There are several options:

- 3 days. The diet should be kept on a minimum amount of meat. Additional products include cucumbers, egg white, cabbage, unsweetened coffee and green tea. The expected plumb line is 2-3 kg.
- 5 days. Assumes the use of 500 g of meat and vegetables. Allowed 100 g of fat-free cottage cheese, 1 unsweetened fruit per day. The prognosis for weight loss is 4-5 kg.
- 7 days. The daily menu is based on lean meat dishes and vegetables. It is allowed to introduce fish or seafood, unsweetened fruits 1-2 times a week. Possible plumb line - 5-6 kg.
- 10 days. The diet is the same as for the weekly duration. Additionally, vitamins should be consumed. You can drop up to 7 kg.


## By type of meat

In the classic version of the diet, it is recommended to alternate several types of meat. Eating only one type of meat contributes to better results. There are several types of meat ration:

- Chicken. You can only use chicken breast, because the remaining parts contain a lot of fat.
- Beef. It is recommended to use fillet, tenderloin stewed or boiled.
- Turkey. The amount of meat should be limited to 0.4 kg, turkey meat contains a lot of phosphorus and cobalt.
- Rabbit. It is recommended to combine rabbit meat with sour fruits, herbs, and spices.

**Additional Ingredients**

To improve the nutritional value, you can supplement the meat diet with one of the food groups:

1. Vegetables. It is recommended to add cucumbers, tomatoes, zucchini, eggplants, onions to the diet.
2. Fruits. Pomegranates, citrus fruits, watermelons, green apples are allowed.
3. Rice. It is permissible to consume 100 g of steamed long-grain or brown rice.
4. Milk products. Low-fat lactic acid products are allowed: cottage cheese, buttermilk, yogurt.

**Meat diet menu:**

In order to comply with calorie content and diet rules, a menu should be drawn up for several days in advance.

| menu on the days | Breakfast | Lunch | Snack | Dinner |
|---|---|---|---|---|
| 1 | 2 boiled eggs; greenery. | beef stew with spices. tea. | grapefruit juice; baked cherry tomatoes. | boiled chicken breast; spinach. |
| 2 | protein omelet; black coffee. | vegetable broth; steamed chicken. | natural yoghurt without additives. | grilled beef with herbs and tomatoes; Orange juice. |
| 3 | lettuce leaves; boiled beef. | a portion of steamed rice; grilled chicken breast. | white cabbage salad and cucumber. | baked turkey fillet; grilled eggplants. |

## Contraindications

Meat is a rough, heavy food. Its excessive use for a long time has a bad effect on the digestive tract. Meat diet for weight loss is prohibited in the presence of:

- gastritis;
- peptic ulcer;
- tendency to constipation;
- intestinal atony;
- kidney pathologies;
- gallstone disease.

# Prana diet

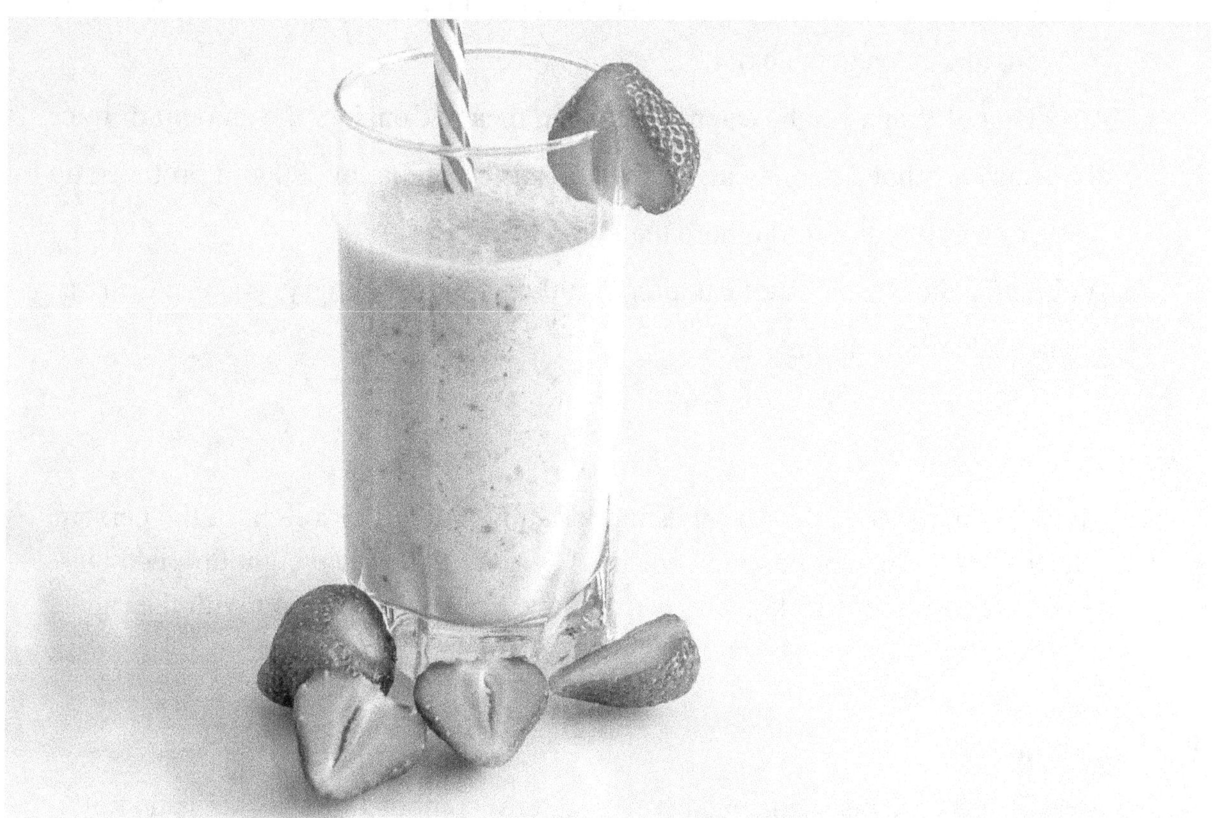

## Prana diet by day

This is a popular variation of the Ducan technique. The Prana diet is considered sparing and does not require serious menu adjustments. The author of the diet was the doctor and scientist Yakov Marshak. After much research, he created a unique protein shake that formed the basis of the Prana two-week diet.

**The essence of the method of losing weight on protein cocktails**

The diet for two weeks according to the Prana system is based on soluble balanced cocktails - sources of vitamins, minerals, protein. The formula of the product is unique, since it gradually reveals all the beneficial properties of the components. Pranic nutrition has the following characteristics:

- One cocktail drunk is equal to a full meal. 1 serving of the drink (30 g of dry powder per 200 ml of water) contains 125 kcal. So much is needed to keep the body running.
- The amount of water you drink per day is at least 2.5 liters.
- Cocktails should be combined with simple foods.
- You need to eat 3 times a day. You need to eat in a relaxed atmosphere. All fried, smoked, high-glycemic foods (mayonnaise and sauces, alcohol, smoked meats) are excluded. The diet should be enriched with fresh natural products (fruits, herbs, chicken, turkey, vegetables).
- A serving of Prana can be eaten in between meals. Consider the amount of trace elements consumed per day and strive for this combination: 90 g of proteins, up to 120 g of carbohydrates, no more than 65 g of fat.
- While on a diet, you cannot eat after 18:00. If you feel hungry, you can drink a Prana cocktail for dinner.

**Diet results**

The amount of lost kg  on  a diet depends individually, the initial weight of the person, respect for rules, regime. On the Prana nutrition system, the body weight dropped on average in 2 weeks is about 15 kg. You can achieve a sustainable result with the right way out of their diet.

**Protein shakes**

Prana food products are distinguished by their natural composition. Cocktails do not contain preservatives, gluten, mercury, sugar. They also do not contain genetically modified foods, heavy metals, nitrates. The composition includes:

- complex of proteins;

- ginger;
- pine nut;
- soy protein;
- phospholipids;
- pectin (apple);
- lecithin;
- flaxseed flour;
- vitamins;
- black pepper extract;
- minerals;
- essential fatty acids,
- magnesium;
- lactulose;
- erythritol sugar substitute.

## Peculiarities of Prana food drinks:

- wide choice of flavors (soups, berry mix, milk dessert);
- balanced environmentally friendly composition;
- it only takes a few minutes to prepare a drink.

## Advantages and Disadvantages of Prana

Nutrition Diet for 14 days according to the Prana system has the following advantages:

- quickly saturates the stomach;
- launches the body cleaning mechanism;
- helps to lose weight;
- makes a person more energetic;
- speeds up metabolism;
- rejuvenates the body;
- has a beneficial effect on the nervous system;
- helps to maintain physical performance;
- lowers blood sugar;
- heals the intestines;

- cheers up;
- reduces the risk of oncology, diabetes, cardiovascular diseases;
- suitable for vegetarians;
- helps fight food addiction;
- can be used for weight gain and muscle mass.

Doctors do not recommend the Prana diet to pregnant and lactating women, since the effect of cocktails on a child has not been studied. The diet is contraindicated for people with pathologies such as:

- oncology;
- stomach ulcer, gastritis;
- diabetes;
- bulimia, anorexia;
- disorders of the kidneys, liver.

There are no obvious shortcomings in pranic nutrition, but when switching to a dietary diet, the following sensations may disturb for some time:

- apathy (indifference), bad mood, depression;
- feeling of hunger (in the early days of the diet);
- weakness, slight dizziness.

## Stages of the 2-week Prana diet

Initially, the 2-week pranic for weight loss was created for people with critically high body weight. Today, the technique is also used to heal the body with the help of protein cocktails.

*For the result to be positive, adhere to the sequence of stages: starting the diet, exiting it, retention and consolidation.*

## Initial stage

Before losing weight, you need to weigh yourself, measure volumes, calculate BMI (body mass index). Record all results in your food diary. Further indicate even small positive changes. If the BMI is 15-50% more than the norm, then the consumption of BJU per day should not exceed the following indicators:

- carbohydrates - 100-200 g;
- proteins - 70–90 g;
- fats - 65–75 g.

## Diet menu:

1. Breakfast. Low-fat cottage cheese (100 g), oatmeal in water (150 g) or cocktail Prana vanilla, chocolate.
2. Lunch. Any protein food: poultry, fish, eggs (200 g).
3. Snack. Prana cocktail gazpacho, broccoli, porcini mushrooms.
4. Dinner. Vegetable salad with oil dressing, boiled egg or berry cocktail.

## Getting out of the diet

This phase of the Prana diet lasts a month. At the end of the program, do not pounce on food immediately, as the weight will quickly return. Gradually introduce low-fat broths, cereals on the water, fruits, vegetables into the diet. Only in the last week can you dine with boiled meat and salad. Before every snack and main meal, be sure to drink 200 ml of warm water with the addition of lemon juice. Diet:

1. Breakfast. One egg cocktail or omelet with spinach (100 g).
2. Snack (in an hour). Grated boiled carrots with flax seeds (100 g).
3. Lunch. Cocktail (porcini mushrooms, gazpacho).
4. Dinner. Low fat cottage cheese (100 g), lazy cabbage rolls (100 g) or Prana cocktail.

## Consolidation of the result

So that after the diet the dropped kilograms do not return, at least once every 7 days spend a fasting day on fish, cottage cheese, vegetables in combination with cocktails. Refuse sweets, smoked, fatty. If this is difficult, you can, for example, eat a piece of dark chocolate instead of a cake. Banned potatoes, ice cream, honey, alcohol, mayonnaise, polished rice, white flour.

# Egg diet

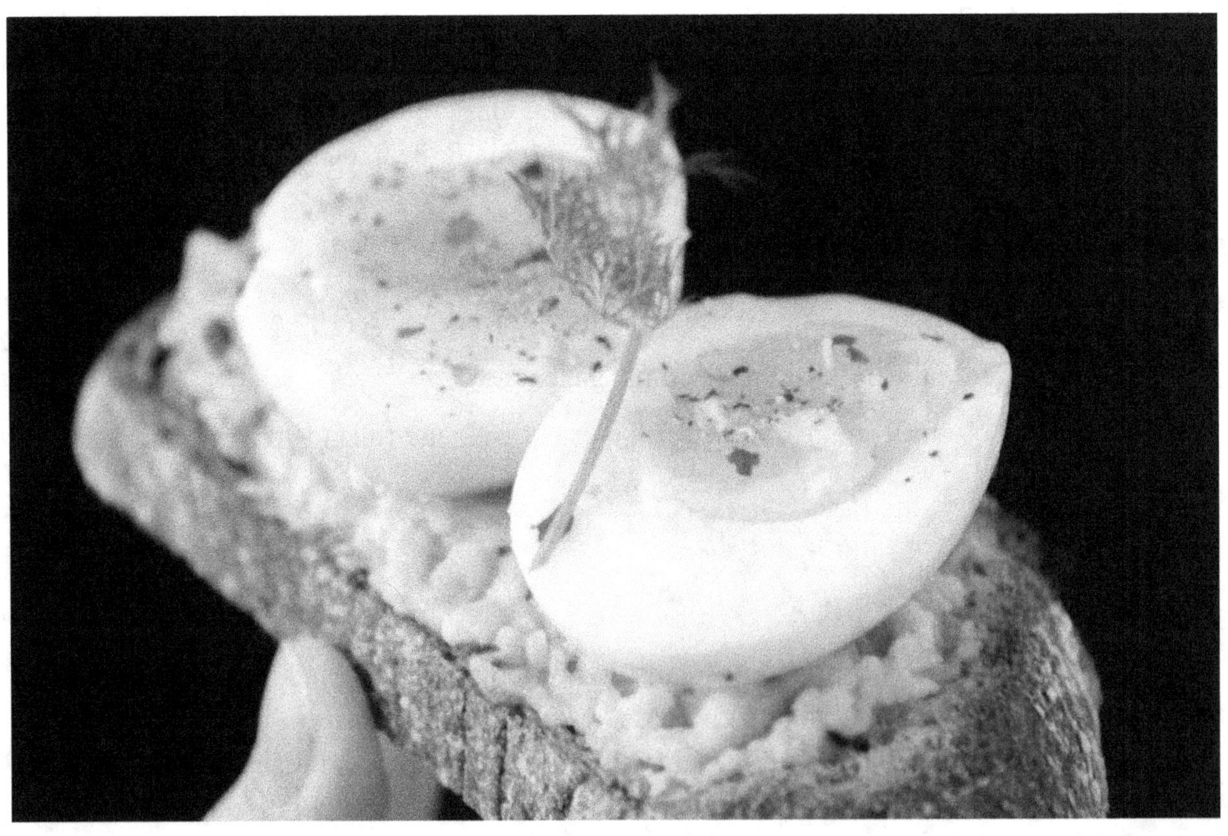

**4 Weeks Egg Diet**

The nutritional system developed by Professor Osama Hamdy was intended for patients with endocrine system problems. It is more difficult for them to lose weight due to hormonal imbalances. A chemical diet helps to change metabolism, use the body's capabilities for weight loss without disrupting its functionality. The system requires endurance from a person, because you need to eat according to a specific menu and adhere of rules, but the result is worth it.

## Features of the egg diet

A carbohydrate-free diet in one month changes the nature of chemical processes in internal systems. The body receives an increased amount of protein, which is not easy to process - it takes energy. There are almost no carbohydrates in the diet menu. There is nowhere to get fast calories. The body begins to consume the fat depot. In the first two weeks, a person eats protein foods, and active weight loss begins. The remaining 14 days are spent on consolidating the result, the menu changes and becomes more diverse.

It is important to strictly follow all dietary guidelines. If you break the rules, don't expect a good result. The frequency of the egg diet is once a year. Don't worry about "bad" cholesterol - eggs are not involved in its formation. The product is quickly digested, providing the body with high-quality protein and vitamins, fats, antioxidants contained in the yolk.

## Principles and rules of nutrition

Strictly adhere to all recommendations. Your goal is to lose weight and rebuild metabolic processes. During the egg diet, follow these rules:

- Eat three times a day. Additional snacks are prohibited. If hunger is annoying, eat a cucumber, carrot, or salad no earlier than 120 minutes after a hearty meal.

- Don't substitute some foods on the menu for others. You cannot shuffle meals, for example, at lunch there is something that is intended for dinner.

- Refuse alcohol. Instead of black tea, you should drink green, herbal tea. The volume of clean water per day is 1.5-2 liters. You can drink soda, but not more than 1 glass a day, a cup of coffee without milk and sugar.

- You cannot eat raw eggs.

- If you do not like boiled eggs, you can bake  or poach them. The main thing is not to use fat when cooking.

- It is forbidden to reduce or increase the serving size. If food weights are not listed in the menu tables, eat until you are full, but do not overeat.

- Cooking methods: boiling in water, stewing, baking, grilling. To make the dishes taste acceptable, they can be seasoned with pepper, salt, onions, and garlic.

- Boil eggs for at least 5 minutes.

## Pros and Cons

The four week egg diet has many benefits. If you love the staple of your diet, give your weight loss system an excellent mark:

- Eggs cook quickly. In the second half of the diet, they are replaced by simple and tasty dishes.
- The diet is suitable for those who like physical activity.
- Products from the menu provide satiety for a long time, so diet has little effect on performance.
- When losing weight, fat is burned and muscles are strengthened.
- In a month, you can lose up to 28 kg (with a very large body weight and exercise).
- The body is saturated with amino acids, manganese, iron, zinc, vitamins of group B, A, choline, biotin and others.

Not everyone will like the 4 week egg and grapefruit diet. If you can barely eat a couple of eggs a week, you shouldn't even start losing weight this way. The system also has objective drawbacks:

- For a long time, the body loses some macronutrients - fast carbohydrates and fatty acids. This affects the functionality of the internal systems.
- An imbalance in the diet leads to various ailments. A common problem with low-carb diets is constipation, headaches, exacerbation of kidney disease, etc.
- There is a risk of poisoning with poor-quality eggs. Before cooking, be sure to wash eggs in hot water or disinfect them with special preparations.

## Permitted products

The list is not too long, but the monotony and strictness of the diet is the key to success. Eating according to a certain menu discipline, makes you change your eating habits. An egg diet for 4 weeks allows you to consume the following products:

- industrial and farm chicken eggs;
- chicken, skinless turkey, beef, veal;
- fat-free cottage cheese 0-5%, hard or soft cheese up to 17% fat;
- all vegetables except potatoes: courgettes, eggplants, squash, carrots, green beans,

tomatoes, bell peppers, young peas, onions, garlic, etc.;

- fruits: in priority grapefruits, oranges; it is allowed to eat tangerines, apricots, peaches, watermelons, apples, pears, pineapples.

## List of prohibited foods

The egg diet for a month does not tolerate violations and the launching of outsider products. You cannot eat semi-finished products, store sauces, margarine, dishes seasoned with synthetic spices, bakery and confectionery products. A taboo is introduced on such harmless products for a thin person:

- lamb, pork;
- meat offal: liver, kidneys, lungs, heart;
- grapes, bananas, mangoes, dates, figs, melons;
- potatoes;
- fat sour cream, cream, homemade cottage cheese, milk;
- butter;
- fat;
- fatty fish.

## A detailed menu of the egg diet for 4 weeks

For four weeks, you need to eat according to the diet idicated in the tables. If the result of losing weight does not satisfy you, repeat the menu of the first and last seven days.

- The breakfast is the same for each day
- Lunches and dinners are more varied. If the amount is not listed, eat until you are full.

## Breakfast

2 hard-boiled or soft-boiled eggs, ½ a grapefruit or orange.

## First week diet:

| Day | Lunch | Dinner |
| --- | --- | --- |
| 1 | Any fruit allowed. | Beef or chicken cooked in any permitted manner. |
| 2 | Chicken, tomato, medium-sized orange. | Vegetable salad, 2 eggs, toast, orange / grapefruit. |

| 3 | Medium tomato, toast, hard cheese. | Chicken breast or beef. |
|---|---|---|
| 4 | Fruit. | Lean meat, fresh vegetable salad. |
| 5 | 2 boiled eggs, stewed vegetables: carrots, peas, zucchini. | Boiled or grilled shrimp / fish, lettuce, medium grapefruit / orange. |
| 6 | Fruit. | Meat, vegetable salad. |
| 7 | Chicken thighs or drumsticks, vegetables, orange. | Boiled / steamed vegetables. |

In the second week, the composition and volume of breakfast do not change. The menu is becoming less diverse - the overweight continues to be hit.

**Second week diet**

| Day | Lunch | Dinner |
|---|---|---|
| 1 | Lettuce, meat. | 2 eggs, lettuce, grapefruit. |
| 2 | **Duplicates the ration of the first day.** | |
| 3 | Grilled / boiled lean meat, cucumber salad without salt and dressing. | 2 eggs, grapefruit. |
| 4 | 2 eggs, boiled vegetables, cottage cheese. | A couple of eggs. |
| 5 | Meat, 2-3 tomatoes. | A couple of eggs. |
| 6 | Meat, 2-3 tomatoes, grapefruit. | Fruit salad without dressing. |

| 7 | Skinless chicken, boiled vegetables, 1 grapefruit. | The same as for lunch. |

In the third week of the egg diet, you will feel a little relief, because the diet will become less strict. All seven days of permitted foods can be eaten without restrictions in volume.

**The diet of the week #3**:

| Day | Products |
| --- | --- |
| 1 | Permitted fruits. |
| 2 | Boiled vegetables, fresh vegetable salads. |
| 3 | Fruits, vegetables. |
| 4 | Fish, lettuce, fresh cabbage, boiled vegetables. |
| 5 | Chicken, fresh vegetables. |
| 6 | Any single fruit. |
| 7 | Any kind of fruit. |

The four-week diet is coming to an end, and the menu becomes even more varied. During these seven days, you gradually return to your normal diet.

**Menu of the last week:**

| Day | Food for the day |
| --- | --- |
| 1 | ¼ boiled chicken without skin or 400 g of other grilled meat, 3 fresh tomatoes, 4 cucumbers, can of canned tuna in its own juice, toast, grapefruit. |
| 2 | 200 g meat, 4 cucumbers, 3 tomatoes, toast, grapefruit, apple / pear. |
| 3 | 300 g boiled vegetables, 2 tomatoes, 2 cucumbers, 1 tbsp. cereal curd, toast, grapefruit. |
| 4 | ½ boiled skinless chicken, cucumber, 3 tomatoes, toast, grapefruit. |

| 5 | May lettuce, tomato 3, 2 boiled eggs, grapefruit. |
|---|---|
| 6 | 2 boiled chicken fillets, toast, 2 cucumbers, 2 tomatoes, 120 g of cottage cheese, 1 glass of buttermilk, grapefruit. |
| 7 | Can of tuna, 200 g of boiled vegetables, 2 cucumbers, 2 tomatoes, 1 tbsp. cottage cheese, toast, grapefruit. |

## Correct way out of the diet

The last week in the system of Osama Hamdy is the beginning of the exit. The stomach is already accustomed to small portions of food, and you began to eat in moderation. At the end of the diet, continue to eat small amounts, gradually introducing cereals, previously prohibited fruits, cheeses, meat and potatoes into the diet. For the first 2-3 weeks, do not eat sugar and all meals containing it. Add fatty foods to the menu very slowly so as not to rip off the pancreas. Eat fatty fish like mackerel, sardines, and sea trout for lunch once a week.

For sweet tooth, until 12:00, can eat 1-2 tsp a couple of times in a week - honey, 1 cube of dark chocolate, toast with nut butter, dates or figs. Don't refuse eggs and citrus fruits right away. Reduce their amount every day. Be sure to drink at least 2 liters of still mineral or filtered water. Alcohol is still banned. After the egg diet, it is optimal to switch to proper nutrition or the -60 system.

## Side Effects

4 week egg diet is not as harmless as it might seem. It is accompanied by unpleasant conditions (not everyone has it):

- nervousness and irritability - associated with a lack of carbohydrates in the diet;
- general poor health, lethargy - a consequence of low-carb nutrition;
- headache due to increased stress on the kidneys;
- flatulence - a consequence of poor tolerance to fruits, some vegetables, egg feeding;
- constipation - occurs due to a high-protein diet and a small amount of fiber in the diet;
- odor from the mouth - formed due to the use of eggs, which, when digested, emit an unpleasant odor;

- heartburn - arises from the frequent use of citrus fruits;
- brittle nails, hair - a consequence of a lack of vitamins, minerals;
- rashes, itching - citrus fruits and eggs are strong allergens.


## Contraindications

The egg-orange diet for 4 weeks is not suitable for everyone because of the specific diet. Contraindications to the weight loss system of Osama Hamdiy:

- pregnancy;
- diseases of the stomach and intestines: gastritis, ulcers, heartburn, flatulence, enterocolitis;
- diseases of the liver, pancreas;
- intolerance to chicken eggs;
- citrus allergy;
- diseases of the heart and blood vessels;
- period after a long illness, weakened immunity.


# 7 petal diet

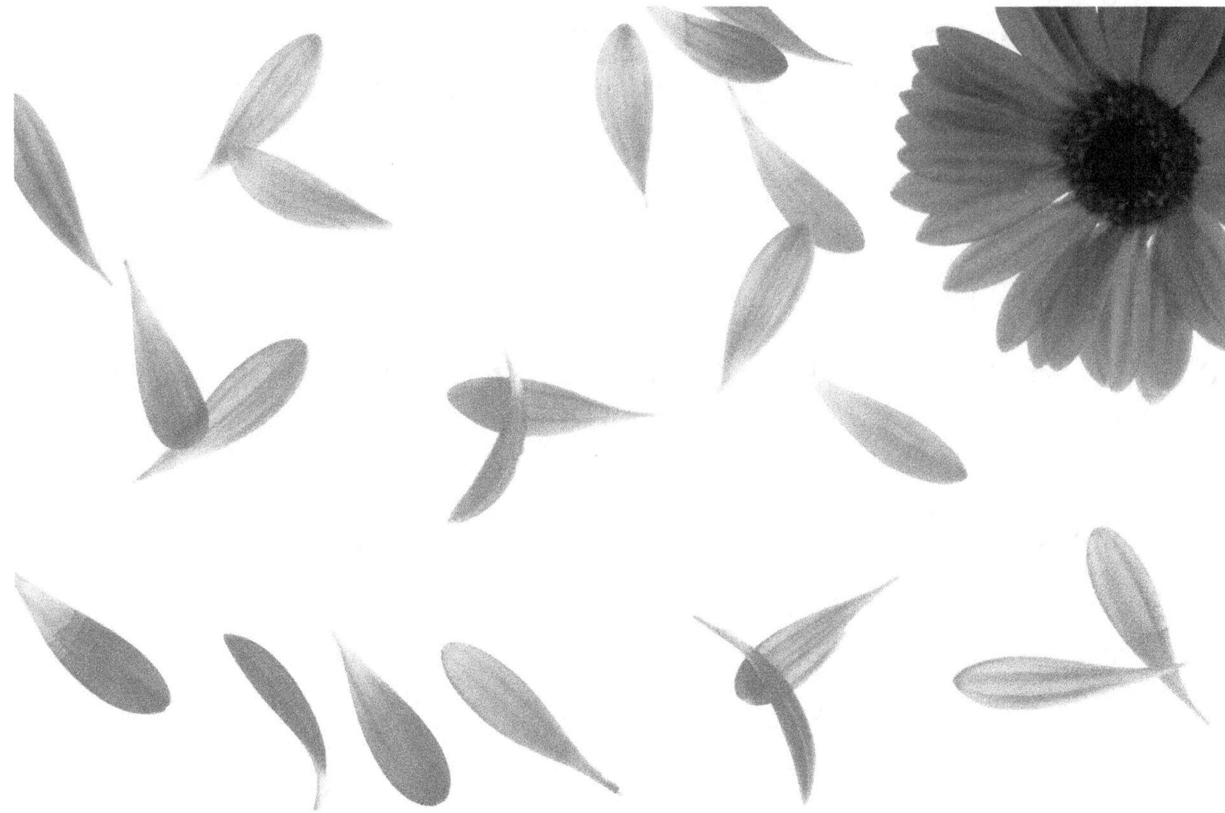

Many women need to limit their food to maintain a beautiful figure. If you belong to this category and want to lose weight quickly, the nutrition system will help "7 petal". This diet is very effective and very popular. Before you dieting, it is recommended to consult with your doctor and find out if it will harm you.

## What is the diet 7-petal

The nutritional system with such an intriguing name was developed by Swedish nutritionist Anna Johansson. The basis of the "7-petal" diet - is the alternation of six mono-diets, which replace each other in succession. Each has 24 hours. The entire weight loss cycle takes a week, during this period it takes 3-5 kg. The diet resembles a game, because a person who plans to follow it is first asked to draw a daisy with six petals and sign each of them in the following sequence:

1. Fish.
2. Vegetable.
3. Chicken.
4. Cereal.
5. Curd.
6. Fruit.

The petals symbolize every day and what to eat. It is recommended to cut the flower and attach it to the refrigerator for more motivation. Having held out each new stage, it is necessary to tear off one petal or add on it how many kilograms you managed to lose. Visualization of the results helps to transfer weight loss much easier.

**How it works**

The 7 Petal Diet works in several ways. The three fundamental principles are:

1.  Protein-carbohydrate alternation. This makes the diet so effective. The first, third, fifth days are protein. The second, fourth, and sixth are carbohydrates. This approach helps to deceive the body. It begins to use up his subcutaneous fat stores, thereby reducing weight. Carbohydrate days are created to avoid "energy" starvation. Fats will enter the body in minimal quantities from chicken, fish, cottage cheese. So, nutrition remains complete and balanced.

2.  Changing daily mono-diets. A uniform diet throughout the day ensures rapid weight loss. This approach to weight loss has been proven to be the most effective.

3.  Separate food. According to the rules, it is forbidden to use products that are not compatible with each other. Incompatible foods have been shown to slow down digestive processes. The incoming fats, carbohydrates and proteins do not have time to be digested, turning into deposits. By following the Seven Petals Diet, you will be eating separately, so you will lose weight quickly.

Each day of the diet has its own functional purpose. How nutrition works during each of them on the body:

1.  Fish. Day of saturation of the body with protein, omega-3 fatty acids. The metabolism is stimulated. You can eat 0.3-0.5 kg of fish or seafood. Dishes can be stewed, boiled, baked.

2.  Vegetables. The body is cleansed. Saturation is provided by starchy vegetable carbohydrates. You can eat up to one and a half kilograms of raw vegetables. Potatoes, canned corn, and peas are prohibited.

3.  Chicken. Day of saturation of the body with energy. You can eat up to half a kilogram of skinless chicken breast. It can be steamed, boiled, or baked.

4.  Cereal. Day of high energy and body fat expenditure. It is allowed to eat up to 300 g of cereals. It is recommended to choose wild or brown rice, oatmeal,

buckwheat. Cereals are rich in vitamins, vegetable protein, starchy carbohydrates and trace elements.

5.  Curd. Day of rejuvenation of the body and a large plumb line. It is allowed to drink fermented milk products or milk and eat up to 0.5 kg of cottage cheese (all fat-free). This will saturate the body with essential amino acids, bacteria, and easily digestible proteins.

6.  Fruit. There is a strong acceleration of metabolism. It is allowed to eat up to 1.5 kg of fruit per day. In the morning, you can take sweets (banana, grapes), the rest of the time - with a low sugar content. Fruits are rich in organic acids, polysaccharides, vitamins and minerals. They can be eaten raw or baked. Can be seasoned with lemon zest, cinnamon, vanilla, cardamom. It is allowed to drink freshly squeezed fruit juices (2-3 glasses).

7.  The seventh day is hungry, unloading. You need to stay on the water for a day (2.5 liters).

**Advantages and Disadvantages**

To decide whether or not to follow the 7-petal diet, you need to understand its pros and cons. The advantages of the food system include:

- 7-petal diet is not accompanied by weakness, a constant feeling of hunger;
- provides real and quick weight loss;
- short duration;
- physical activity is allowed;
- the body receives all the vitamins, trace elements and other substances that it needs.

There are also many disadvantages of the Seven-Flower power system. Negative points of this diet:

1.  It is not suitable for people with individual intolerance to one or more components.

2.  Eating often and fractionally is inconvenient for people who work, it is better to postpone the diet until vacation.

3.  The Seven-Flower Diet is not suitable for people who have diseases of the stomach, intestines and liver.

**Rules**

The 7-petal diet's food system has a number of requirements that must be followed in order for weight loss to be effective. Sitting on a diet, you must follow these rules:

1. Days are prohibited from swapping. Their sequence is strictly defined, because the effectiveness of the diet is provided by protein-carbohydrate alternation.

2. It is advisable to play sports. Physical activity should be moderate.

3. Dishes cannot be fried. They can be boiled, baked, and steamed. Thesalt is allowed in a minimum amount.

4. There should be five meals a day.

5. If you want to strengthen the effect of the diet and lose even more, you can repeat another cycle in a week.

6. Food should always be chewed slowly and thoroughly.

7. Any foods containing sugar are excluded. You cannot eat sweets, flour.

8. While losing weight, you need to drink a lot of pure non-carbonated water, but before or after a meal. Drinking food is prohibited. Also allowed 1-2 cups of black or green tea or coffee, but no sugar. Alcohol is prohibited.

## Diet menu for every day

If you find it difficult to compose a diet, use a ready-made example. Menu option for the whole week:

| Day of the week | Breakfast | Lunch (snack) | Lunch | Afternoon snack | Dinner |
|---|---|---|---|---|---|
| **Monday** (0.3-0.5 kg of fish or seafood) | 100 g of boiled sea bass fillet (can be replaced with pike perch, hake, cod). | 100 g of baked low-fat fish, seasoned with herbs. | Seafood soup without vegetables. | 100 g steamed fish. | 100 g of boiled pike perch with spices and herbs. |
| **Tuesday** (up to 1.5 kg of vegetables) | Grated carrots or turnips. | Eggplant and zucchini stew. | Stewed cabbage. | Steamed carrots and beets. | Any raw vegetables. |
| **Wednesday** (up to 0.5 kg of chicken) | Boiled breast. | Fillet baked in foil with dill. | Chicken broth with pieces of meat and herbs. | Grilled fillet. | Boiled breast. |
| **Thursday** (up to 300 g of cereals) | Any cereal porridge on the water. | Hercules. | Rice porridge. | Oatmeal. | Buckwheat with herbs. |
| **Friday** (up to 0.5 kg of cottage cheese) | Low-fat cottage cheese with natural yogurt. | Cottage cheese 1% fat, a glass of milk. | Cottage cheese 5% fat. | Cottage cheese with buttermilk. | Low fat cottage cheese. |
| **Saturday** (up to 1.5 kg of fruits and berries) | 2 green apples. | Banana. | Grapefruit or orange, a small bunch of grapes. | 3 kiwi. | 2 red apples. |

| **Sunday** | Still water (2.5 l) |

## Rules for withdrawing from the diet

It is necessary to follow certain recommendations so that the lost kilograms do not return. How to get out of the Seven:

1. Eat foods from your diet, but you may not comply with the daily restrictions.
2. Gradually increase the calorie content of the daily diet to 1800 kcal.
3. Do not eat smoked, fried, fatty, semi-finished products, fast food. It is also better to abstain from carbonated drinks.
4. Try to consume more protein and less carbohydrates.
5. Limit yourself to sweets and pastries.

## Contraindications

7-petal is a tough diet that some people are strictly forbidden to follow. Before getting on it, be sure to consult with your doctor to make sure that you have no health problems. Contraindications to diet are:

- pregnancy;
- chronic diseases of the gastrointestinal tract;
- lactation period;
- hormone therapy;
- anemia;
- chemotherapy;
- diabetes.

**Recipes**

To keep the diet easier, you need to come up with new dishes, because five times a day to eat the same will get boring. It will be easy to create a menu with a wide range of permitted foods. If you connect your imagination and try to experiment, then provide yourself with a varied diet on a diet. Explore several recipes suitable for Seven Blossom.

**Baked fruit salad**

- Time: half an hour.
- Servings Per Container: 4 Persons.
- Calorie content of the dish: 41 kcal (per 100 g).
- Purpose: 6th petal, supper.
- Cuisine: European.
- Difficulty: easy.

A light fruit salad is a great dinner option for the last day of your diet with the most delicious menu. It is very easy to prepare it. This dish is a storehouse of vitamins and nutrients. According to the recipe, the salad includes apples, oranges, pears, kiwi and dried apricots, but you can slightly change the composition by replacing the listed fruits with other savory ones. You will spend only half an hour on cooking.

Ingredients:

- apples - 4 pcs .;
- dried apricots - 6 pcs.;
- oranges - 4 pcs.;
- kiwi - 2 pcs.;
- pears - 2 pcs.

Cooking method:

1. Pour dried apricots with boiled water. Leave it on for 5 minutes.
2. Peel oranges, kiwi.
3. Cut all fruit into small cubes. Stir. You can add a little cinnamon or vanilla.
4. Place the fruit on a baking sheet, greased with a little vegetable oil.
5. Bake in an oven preheated to 180 degrees for a quarter of an hour.

**Curd mousse**

- Time: 20 min.
- Servings Per Container: 1 person.
- Caloric content of the dish: 74 kcal (per 100 g).
- Purpose: 5 petal, breakfast.
- Cuisine: European.
- Difficulty: easy.

The curd day of the diet is difficult to tolerate, because it involves a monotonous diet. You can remedy the situation by making a light and nutritious mousse with the following recipe. A little honey is added to the slimming dish, so it is better to eat it for breakfast. In addition to cottage cheese, milk goes into the mousse, but according to the rules of the diet, this is permissible. Cooking is very simple, absolutely anyone can handle it.

Ingredients:

- low fat cottage cheese - 125 g;
- cinnamon - a pinch;
- honey - 0.5 tsp;
- milk with a low percentage of fat - 50 ml.

Cooking method:

1. Put cottage cheese in a deep container.
2. Pour in milk, add honey, and cinnamon.
3. Beat the food with a blender until smooth.

**Cream of tomato soup**

- Time: 40 min.
- Servings Per Container: 1 person.
- Calorie content of the dish: 55 kcal (per 100 g).
- Purpose: 2 petals, lunch.

- Cuisine: European.
- Difficulty: easy.

Tomato soup is easy to cook and is perfect for lunch on the second vegetable day of the diet. Such a dish is very healthy and it is recommended to leave it in your diet even after you finish eating according to the rules of the 7 petals. The puree soup turns out to be very thick and aromatic, a little garlic and basil are added to it. You can salt and pepper the dish, but in moderation.

Ingredients:

- tomatoes - 250 g;
- garlic - 1 clove;
- onion - 1 small head;
- pepper, basil, salt - to taste.

Cooking method:

1. Peel and finely chop the onion, garlic.
2. Pour some water into a saucepan. Cook the garlic and onion for 10 minutes.
3. Peel the tomatoes, cut into cubes. Place in a saucepan.
4. Cook for another 5 minutes over low heat.
5. Pour in some water, bring to a boil. Cook for 10 minutes.
6. Turn it off, let it brew a little.
7. Add spices and puree with a blender. Add some basil.

# Afterword

A consultation with a nutritionist will help you to start the process of losing weight competently, who will individually find out the reason for weight gain and suggest a suitable method for reducing.

When visiting a dietitian, be honest. Don't hide your nutritional weaknesses and play down your weight problems. This makes no sense - you are only deceiving yourself, and for the doctor, misinformation will only become an obstacle to the selection of objective methods of losing weight.

Perhaps the existing eating habits will be severely criticized by the nutritionist. Be prepared for the fact that some products, regardless of your health condition, will tell you to give up right away.

After consulting with a nutritionist, you will find foods high in fiber and protein in your kitchen. Fresh fruits, vegetables and herbs should become permanent on your table. As a side dish, you need to choose complex carbohydrates. Ideal in this regard would be buckwheat, brown or wild rice, peas and soybeans. The best sources of protein would be dietary turkey or chicken breast, lamb, rabbit meat, or lean sea fish. If the patient has the opportunity, it is worth enriching their diet with seafood, as they contain a lot of magnesium, iodine, calcium, phosphorus and molybdenum, which are important for maintaining optimal metabolism. In addition, most seafood is low in calories. Special attention should be paid to berries, citrus fruits, spinach, celery and lettuce. These foods can help make any meal less nutritious and increase your metabolic rate.

Experts recommend paying special attention to drinking water, which is necessary to accelerate metabolism, break down fats, and remove toxins. It is advisable to drink a liter for every 30 kilograms of weight.

## Advise of food experts

**Nutritional advice from nutritionists:**

- give up the fast food;
- eat fruits, vegetables;
- be sure to have breakfast;
- exclude soda from the diet.
- limit any sweets;
- exclude flour, fatty foods;
- arrange fasting days;
- remove late dinner.

**Right weight loss**

- to know what result you want to get in kilograms or subtracted centimeters;
- to combine weight loss techniques with the capabilities, characteristics of the body;
- to draw up an action plan, determine the timing.
- to compliance with the calorie content of food no more than 2500 kcal per day;
- to exclusion of large amounts of vegetable fats;
- restriction of potatoes, cereals;
- integreat of fermented milk products, natural juices;
- to eat rye bread.

**To lose weight properly**

- reasonable weight loss - no more than a kilogram per week;
- you cannot exhaust yourself with hunger - you can quickly restore what was lost;
- it is important not to overeat;
- reduce the calorie content of food due to cooking technology, exclude frying, prefer steamed, boiled dishes.
- eat often, in small portions;
- part of the diet should be proteins, the rest - slow carbohydrates;
- eat foods that help break down fats - grapefruit, celery;
- use bran for food - fiber contributes to the satiety effect, helps to remove toxins;
- use fermented milk products;
- walk daily;
- replace sugar with honey;

**In addition**

- eat more greens, vegetables;
- apply vitamin complexes;
- on holidays, do not eat everything - try no more than 3 dishes.
- use quality products for food;
- eat meat and cereals for lunch;
- in the evening, eat baked vegetables, scrambled eggs, seafood;
- exclude sausages, sweets, mayonnaise;
- limit salt and foods containing it;
- use pumpkin, linseed oil in cooking;
- eat protein foods - fish, lean meat, poultry;
- do not overeat under stress.